WO 190
SER.
S4264

WITHDRAWN

Positioning patients for surgery

**Library
Knowledge Spa
Treliske
Truro
TR3 6HD**
01872 256444

This item is to be returned on or before the last date
stamped below. To renew items please contact the library

21 DAY LOAN

0 8 OCT 2004   RETURNED
RETURNED   - 3 JUL 2007
RETURNED
1 0 JUN 2009
0 2 MAY 2006   RETURNED
0 9 OCT 2006   1 7 NOV 2009
RETURNED   0 8 RETURNED 2012
2 4 JAN 2007 RETURNED 2015
RETURNED   2 9 JUN 2016
3 0 MAR 2007   RETURNED

D1354243

Positioning patients for surgery

Chris Servant, BSc(Hons), MB, BS, FRCS

Orthopaedic Specialist Registrar
Royal United Hospital
Bath, UK

Shaun Purkiss, MS, FRCS(Gen)

Senior Lecturer
Royal London Hospital
Whitechapel
London, UK

With contributions from

John Hughes

Senior Operating Department Assistant
Royal United Hospital
Bath, UK

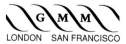

LONDON   SAN FRANCISCO

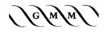

Greenwich Medical Media
4th Floor, 137 Euston Road,
London
NW1 2AA

© 2002

870 Market Street, Ste 720
San Francisco
CA 94109, USA

ISBN   1 84110 052 8

First published 2002

Apart from any fair dealing for the purposes of research or private study, or criticism or review, as permitted under the UK Copyright Designs and Patents Act 1988, this publication may not be reproduced, stored, or transmitted, in any form or by any means, without the prior permission in writing of the publishers, or in the case of reprographic reproduction only in accordance with the terms of the licences issued by the appropriate Reproduction Rights Organisations outside the UK. Enquiries concerning reproduction outside the terms stated here should be sent to the publishers at the London address printed above.

The rights of Chris Servant, Shaun Purkiss and John Hughes to be identified as authors of this work have been asserted by them in accordance with the Copyright Designs and Patents Act 1988.

The publisher makes no representation, express or implied, with regard to the accuracy of the information contained in this book and cannot accept any legal responsibility or liability for any errors or omissions that may be made.

A catalogue record for this book is available from the British Library.

www.greenwich-medical.co.uk

Distributed worldwide by Plymbridge Distributors Ltd and in the USA by Jamco Distribution

Typeset by Phoenix Photosetting, Chatham, Kent
Printed by The Alden Group, Oxford

Contents

Acknowledgements

The authors would like to thank the following for their help in the preparation of this book:

John Hughes, Senior Operating Department Assistant, Royal United Hospital, Bath

Caroline Sherwood, Trainee Operating Department Assistant, Royal United Hospital, Bath

Keith Bolton, Sales Engineer, Maquet, UK

Joseph Widowski, Senior Operating Department Assistant, Southmead Hospital, Bristol

Introduction

The positioning of patients for surgical operations is often omitted or mentioned only briefly in operative texts. More attention is usually afforded to the description of the surgical approach and the surgical procedure itself. However, accurate set-up is obligatory. Without it the rest of the operation is likely to be more challenging or even hazardous. Each operative position represents an agreement between the surgeon and the anaesthetist. This agreement should not be a competitive exercise, as the deal struck by both practitioners considers the safety of the patient as the utmost priority.

The surgeon requires an adequate area in which to perform the operation. The position chosen should provide accessibility to the surgical field that remains stable for the duration of the operation. The anaesthetist has similar requirements. They may be administering a local, regional or a general anaesthetic, and they must have access to the patient after the surgery has started. The position chosen, therefore, must allow the anaesthetist the ability to continue the anaesthetic, administer intravenous fluids and provide access to monitor the patient. It is both the surgeon's and anaesthetist's responsibility, with support and often guidance from allied health care workers, that the risks from a particular position are reduced to an absolute minimum.

This book has been designed to guide the approach of all theatre personnel in how to position a patient for a procedure in general and orthopaedic surgery. It is a guide, as local and individual practitioners' preferences vary. No position is entirely safe and none are set in stone. A healthy communication between all theatre staff is in the patient's interest, both during the process of achieving the operative position and afterwards, to discuss potential improvements and modifications. These should be introduced if they have the potential to eliminate risk. A continuous reappraisal of any technique used is essential in maintaining standards, and this will improve the overall safety for patients.

In short, correct positioning leads to safer and easier surgery.

Please note that in the text of this book:

- Descriptions and diagrams relate to the right side being operated upon. For the left side the position should be mirrored.
- Only the more commonly used surgical positions are described.
- The set-up described for a particular position may not be the only way of setting up a patient, but it is known to be a safe and successful method.
- More than one position may work for any one surgical approach.

Aims of good patient positioning

• Patient comfort	—particularly if general anaesthesia is not employed
• Patient dignity	
• Patient stability and security	—during and after transfer on to the operating table
• Maintenance of normal physiology	—e.g. minimal interference with circulation
• Protection of important structures	—e.g. protection of nerves
• Ease of surgical access	
• Ease of anaesthetic access	
• Ease of access for theatre equipment	—e.g. image intensifier, operating microscope
• Avoidance of complications	—e.g. pressure sores, excessive bleeding

Medicolegal considerations

"I will follow that system of regimen which, according to my ability and judgement, I consider for the benefit of my patients, and abstain from whatever is deleterious and mischievous."

(The Oath of Hippocrates, fifth century BC)

"Doctors must practise good standards of clinical care and ensure that patients are not put at unnecessary risk."

(General Medical Council: Good Medical Practice, 1998)

General considerations

The operating theatre is a hazardous environment for all persons. When a patient is given a general anaesthetic they lose all ability to protect and fend for themselves. As a consequence, all staff within the operating department must take over this protective function, and they have a responsibility to ensure that every patient is safe. Good clinical practice is required to ensure that the safety of all manoeuvres performed in theatre (such as a transfer or the achievement of a surgical position) is constantly appraised and audited to maintain good standards.

The surgeon is ultimately responsible for patient safety in this environment, and is the usual focus for medicolegal issues when things go wrong. The achievement of an adequate and safe surgical position to perform an operation is only one small part of their overall responsibility. The surgeon usually takes an active role in positioning a patient as it can facilitate the operation. It is appropriate to outline the surgeon's other responsibilities to a particular patient undergoing surgery.

These include ensuring that:

- a preoperative interview with the patient has occurred and appropriate preoperative investigations have been performed including marking the patient's operative site (It is becoming clearer that the senior surgeon involved in the patient's care is required to obtain adequate informed consent.)
- the correct patient is being operated upon
- it is the correct operation for the patient
- the correct side is being operated upon
- appropriate support services are available for the operation e.g. blood products, radiological facility and personnel if required.

Responsibility

Doctors have a duty to maintain a good standard of practice and to care and show respect for their patients. In the operating theatre, the surgeon and the anaesthetist must work as a team to ensure their patient's well-being before, during and after an operation.

In relation to the positioning of a patient for surgery, all theatre personnel must:

- treat every patient politely and considerately
- ensure the comfort of the patient

- respect a patient's dignity
- avoid complications (*primum non nocere* – first do no harm).

It is not the aim of this book to consider other medicolegal issues related to surgical treatment, such as informed consent.

Patient comfort

Patient comfort is particularly pertinent when general anaesthesia is not being used, but even when the patient is unconscious it is good practice to treat the patient as if he or she were conscious. The surgical position should look comfortable, and it may be sensible to rehearse the surgical position prior to anaesthesia to make sure it is indeed comfortable.

Patient dignity

Patients often feel at their most vulnerable in an operating theatre. Respecting a patient's dignity requires the following:

- Minimising exposure of the patient
- Avoiding the use of inappropriate behaviour, including speech, irrespective of the conscious state of the patient.

Patient safety

Essentially, this requires the avoidance of complications, such as:

- pressure sores
- nerve injuries
- spinal injuries
- cardiorespiratory complications
- diathermy burns
- tourniquet sores.

These will be discussed further in the following section.

Other considerations

Operating tables

Operating tables (especially orthopaedic traction tables) vary greatly in how they operate. Therefore, it is advisable for the surgeon, anaesthetist and operating department assistant (ODA) to familiarise themselves with the operation of a table and its relevant attachments before a patient is placed upon it.

Essential characteristics of a good operating table (Figure 1)

- Stable — usually achieved by having a heavy base
- Easily manoeuvrable — mobile tables have some form of lockable castor system
- Highly adjustable — by use of either electro-hydraulic or hand-operated controls, the following adjustments should be possible: height, lateral tilt, head-down (Trendelenburg) and head-up (reverse Trendelenburg) tilt, central break (sitting and jack-knife positions)
- Adaptable — it should be possible to attach a variety of supports, rests and traction extensions; one half of the table should be removable
- Comfortable — soft rubber cushions are removable and easily cleaned
- Radiolucent — a large section should be radiolucent to allow X-ray films or an image intensifier to be used

Table accessories

Arm boards / gutters (Figure 2, Figure 3)
Padded head support / head ring (Figure 4)
Lumbar supports (Figure 5)
Abdominal support (padded cylindrical post) (Figure 6)
Thigh support (with or without condyle supports) (see Figure 80)
Leg holder (for arthroscopy) (see Figure 72)
Cylindrical foot support (Figure 7)
Lithotomy poles
Lloyd-Davies stirrups (Figure 8)
Traction extension pieces (see below)

Clamps, which secure the accessories to the table side-rails
Various shapes and sizes of gel pad
Sandbags
Vacuum mattress

The orthopaedic traction table (Figure 9)

The orthopaedic traction table generally has separate leg supports, which replace the bottom end of the conventional operating table. A central sacral support is also included.

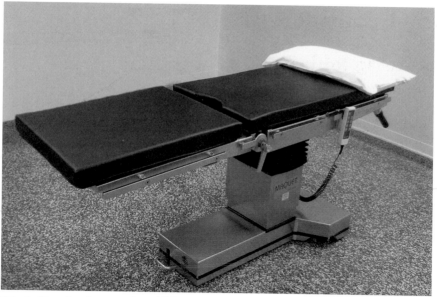

FIG. 1 **Standard operating table**

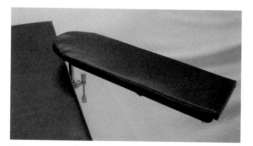

FIG. 2 **Arm board**

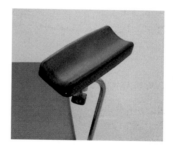

FIG. 3 **Gutter**

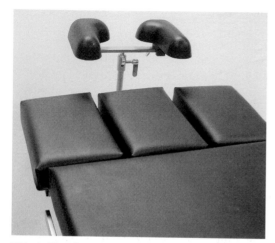

FIG. 4 **Head support**

Once the patient has been transferred on to the operating table, a well-padded perineal post is inserted into an appropriate hole in the table for counter-traction (Figure 10). The patient is then carefully pulled down on to the post such that traction will be applied against the ipsilateral pubic rami.

The legs of the patient are then secured to the traction attachment. The attachment may be a pair of traction arms (which are integral to most traction tables; see Figure 9) or a central traction bar (Figure 11), which can be added once the leg supports have been removed. Both the traction arms and the central traction bar are telescopic horizontal metal bars to which are secured adjustable vertical bars. The patient's leg can then be fixed to the vertical bar by one of a variety of attachments. The leg through which traction is to be applied can be secured to a traction boot (see Figure 59), a traction plate or a traction stirrup (via a traction pin) (see Figure 64). The contralateral leg may be placed either in a traction boot or on a padded gutter.

When placing a patient into position on traction, always hold the patient's leg and move it into position before securing it to the traction extension. Moving the leg after it has been secured to the extension applies considerable leverage to the leg, which may result in an iatrogenic fracture, especially in elderly patients with osteoporotic bones.

Patient transfer

General

Prior to patient transfer (ideally prior to the patient entering the anaesthetic room), the following should be checked:

- The surgeon, anaesthetist and ODA are familiar with the operating table. Operating tables (especially orthopaedic traction tables) vary greatly.
- The operating table is set up correctly. For example, if traction needs to be applied, check that the appropriate traction attachment is attached, and, if image intensification is to be used, ensure that the relevant section of the table is radiolucent.
- The patient's centre of gravity will be centred over the table base when set up in the surgical position (depending on the table design).
- The required table accessories are available.

Transfer on to the operating table should be a co-ordinated, controlled and smooth process. This is made easier if the patient is lying on a canvas undersheet, which can be held in preference to the patient. Ensure that no attachments to the patient, such as drip tubing or catheter bags, are going to become caught up.

There should be one person in charge of the transfer, usually the anaesthetist. Transfer should begin on a pre-agreed count.

If positioning a patient into a complex position, or if there are concerns about a possible spinal injury, make sure the whole team is clear about their role in the transfer process.

The head and neck should be kept in a neutral position.

Transfer devices, such as slides, minimise shearing forces on the skin.

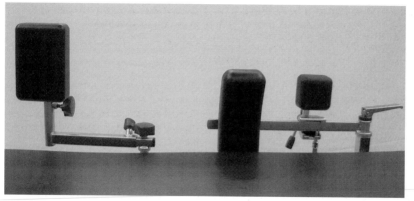

FIG. 5 **A variety of side and lumbar supports**

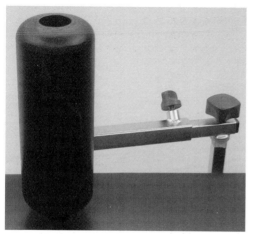

FIG. 6 **Vertical post (abdominal support)**

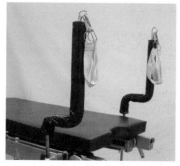

FIG. 8 **Lithotomy poles with Lloyd-Davies stirrups**

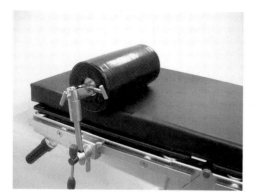

FIG. 7 **Horizontal post (foot support)**

Care of spinal injuries (actual and potential)

In multiply injured patients, in the presence of a spinal injury or if a spinal injury has not been excluded, ensure that the patient's spine is kept aligned in neutral at all times. A semi-rigid cervical collar may be required, and a coordinated transfer on to the operating table is mandatory.

Rheumatoid patients

Cervical instability is a frequent problem in rheumatoid patients. The upper cervical spine tends to be affected and atlanto-axial instability is common. Flexion and extension radiographs of the cervical spine are an essential part of the pre-operative work-up and, in the presence of significant instability, the neck must be protected in a neck collar, and excessive flexion should be avoided peri-operatively.

Securing the patient

After patient transfer, adjustments to the patient's position are made according to the final position required (see the specific descriptions of individual positions).

The patient should be stabilised on the operating table with the use of pillows, beanbags, sandbags or other supports. Certain positions require the use of specific mattresses and table attachments to secure the patient.

Catheters

Ensure that a urinary catheter or other tubing is out of the surgical field, is not going to be pulled during set-up and is secured (e.g. by taping to the operating table).

Effect of patient position on the circulation and respiration

Supine

The ventilation:perfusion ratio is greatest in the dependent parts of both lungs.

Patients with cardiorespiratory disease may become dyspnoeic when lying flat, and they may need to be raised up on pillows into a more tolerable position.

Pregnant patients may become hypotensive when supine as a result of pressure on the inferior vena cava from the pregnant uterus (Supine Hypotensive Syndrome). 20° of right-sided tilt will help relieve the pressure.

Trendelenburg

The ventilation:perfusion ratio is best at the apices (the reverse of the normal upright posture).

Increased pressure on the diaphragm from abdominal contents decreases the compliance of the lungs. Therefore, to achieve adequate ventilation, greater airway pressures are needed, particularly in obese patients.

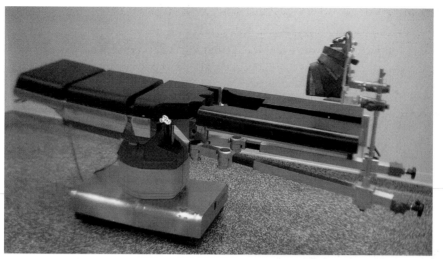

FIG. 9 **An orthopaedic traction table with leg extension pieces, traction arms and traction boots**

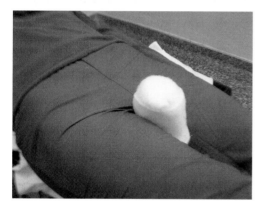

FIG. 10 **Padded perineal post**

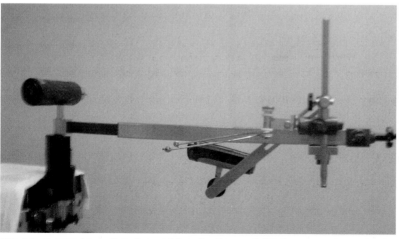

FIG. 11 **Central traction bar with a horizontal thigh support, a traction stirrup and a gutter attached**

Venous return from the lower limbs is increased, but arterial supply may be reduced to below critical levels.

Reverse Trendelenburg (sitting)

Patients with a fixed cardiac output (e.g. valvular heart disease, hypovolaemia) do not tolerate rapid movement from a supine to a more erect position, and they may become hypotensive.

Hypotension may be minimised by gradually changing the patient's position.

Cerebral perfusion is reduced, and this may become critical in the presence of hypotension.

Air embolism is a risk in neurosurgery performed in the sitting position (when the head is above the level of the heart).

Ventilation is easier in an erect or semi-erect position, but hyperventilation may further reduce venous return.

Lateral

The upper lung is less perfused but better ventilated.

Prone

The ventilation:perfusion ratio is best in the anterior portions of the lungs.

The lungs will have less compliance, and greater airway pressures will be required.

Pressure on the abdomen may decrease venous return from the lower extremity and increase the tendency to bleed.

Protection of important structures

Nerves

Nerves are highly vulnerable to traction and pressure. Injuries are an avoidable complication of a surgical operation but, fortunately, they occur rarely. In a series from Spain the estimated incidence was 6 in 2750 patients (Gonzalez A et al, Rev Esp Anesthesiol Reanm 1995 42(3): 100–102) of which 3 (incidence: approximately 1 in 1000) were considered directly related to the surgical position. These injuries, albeit infrequent, are potentially debilitating complications, and they often result in medicolegal action. The most common injuries affect the ulnar and common peroneal nerves, although more centrally placed nerves such as the brachial plexus and the lumbosacral roots can also be affected. The underlying mechanism of injury is believed to be associated with traction and/or compression of the nerve or plexus during the operation. The exact pathophysiological events leading to a neuropathy remain to be established. Ischaemic effects on the nerve are considered important in the development of a neuropathy. The vasa nervosum (the small arteries that travel along the nerve fibres) are fragile, and they can easily thrombose or tear as a result of compression or a traction injury. The subsequent development of local anoxia and accumulation of metabolic products may play a role in the aetiology of nerve dysfunction. The recovery time varies from a few hours to nearly one year. Factors that affect recovery include the severity of the injury and the presence of medical co-morbidity such as diabetes, alcoholism, arteriosclerosis and hypertension. It is usual that the sensory impairment improves before motor function returns.

Cervical spine

The cervical spine should always be protected if there is a recognised cervical spine injury, e.g., following trauma.

Patients with cervical spondylosis, who may develop entrapment neuropathies from extremes of neck position, and patients with rheumatoid arthritis, who may be at risk of suffering an odon toid peg pithing injury to the spinal cord, should be recognised in the preoperative stage. The preoperative interview is essential in identifying these disease processes, and an assessment should be made of the risk that the operative position may precipitate an injury. Preoperative cervical spine radiology will help in assessment and show that this problem was considered should an injury develop. The main source of error is failure to recognise that a potential problem exists. As soon as X-rays have been taken and the potential problem has been identified, this should be communicated to all staff moving and positioning a patient. Occasionally a neck collar or skull traction may be required during anaesthesia.

In a patient with no evidence of cervical spine disease, gentle movement with avoidance of even moderate extremes of angulation or rotation is appropriate.

Brachial plexus

The brachial plexus is derived from the cervical spinal nerves 5–8 and the thoracic spinal nerve 1. The plexus is attached centrally to the bony vertebrae and prevertebral fascia. Distally the plexus is attached to the axillary sheath. The brachial plexus is consequently susceptible to any stretch between these two points. Abduction of the arm above 90° is particularly prone to cause an injury associated with distraction of these two fixed points of the brachial plexus. For example, when positioning patients for surgery on the axilla during an axillary lymphadenectomy, or when the patient is in the lateral position for thoracotomy or kidney surgery and the free arm is held in a gutter and used for i.v. access, there is a tendency to push the limits of arm movements to more than 90° of abduction and flexion. In these instances injuries have been described and, as a consequence, this practice should be avoided.

Lumbo-sacral roots

Traction injuries may occur as a consequence of prolonged hyperflexion of the hip. The lithotomy position used for operations on the perineum is the position primarily associated with this form of injury. As with the brachial plexus, it is important to avoid an angle of more than 90° at the hips.

Common peroneal nerve

Compression of the peroneal nerve is a common problem for patients, and it is particularly prone to occur in the lithotomy and Lloyd-Davies positions. The common peroneal nerve runs around the superior (top) of the lateral (outside) aspect of the fibula in the calf. An injury to this nerve can cause foot inversion and drop from uninhibited action of the opposing muscle groups.

This problem can be avoided by placing the legs outside the lithotomy poles, by using padding over the nerve and by avoiding any pressure on this area of the lower leg.

Ulnar nerve

The ulnar nerve in the arm is prone to injury similarly to the common peroneal nerve. The nerve passes under the medial epicondyle of the humerus at the elbow and is particularly prone to pressure from poorly placed arm restraints and table attachments. This injury should be actively avoided by padding around the elbow in most surgical procedures if this is not the operative site

Summary

Certain nerves, such as the brachial plexus, ulnar nerve and common peroneal nerve, are particularly at risk due to incorrect positioning.

Attention to detail in setting up the patient into the correct position will minimise the potential for peri-operative nerve injury. There should be no undue tension within the neck, upper limbs or lower limbs. In general, a patient should be secured in a position that would seem comfortable if the patient were not anaesthetised.

The head and neck should be kept in as neutral a position as possible, particularly in the presence of an actual or potential cervical spinal injury.

Pressure areas

- Ensure any pressure areas are well-padded to prevent skin breakdown and nerve compression, e.g. areas under a lumbar support, the sacral area, the heels, the greater trochanter, the head of the fibula.
- Suitable padding should be placed under the pelvis, chest, head and nose to allow adequate ventilation when the patient is positioned prone.

Particular care needs to be afforded to patients with delicate skin (e.g. due to old age, steroid use, peripheral oedema, dehydration) or peripheral vascular disease.

Skin breakdown will result in a pressure sore.

Traction injuries

Traction tables pose specific problems with patient positioning:

- Counter-traction is usually provided by a perineal post. This must be well-padded and should rest against the pubic rami on the operative side. It should not press against the external genitalia or the pudendal nerve.
- Care should be exercised in ensuring that the patient is not pulled off the table when positioning the patient or applying traction.
- Patients with delicate skin should be handled carefully and traction should be applied with caution.

Delicate areas

Ensure delicate areas (e.g. perineum, corneas) are protected appropriately.

The corneas are best protected by keeping the eyelids closed during surgery using tape. It is imperative that local pressure on the globe of the eye is avoided at all times as raised pressure or globe injury can result in permanent blindness.

The lips and teeth are susceptible to injury during intubation and general airway management. Endoscopic procedures are also associated with injuries to this area. These may be avoided by being aware of their possibility. Identifying susceptible patients (such as those patients with crowns on their teeth), the use of a mouth guard and appropriate modification of technique for those particularly at risk can all decrease the probability of injury.

Chest

Adequate movement of the chest to enable ventilation is mandatory. Any impediment such as local pressure from, for example, a surgeon's arms and elbows should be avoided. Most positions result in a reduction in ventilation compared with the supine dorsal recumbent position. The prone jack-knife and Trendelenburg positions have particularly adverse effects on ventilatory capacity.

Temperature regulation

In long operations or for certain individuals (e.g. very young, very old, hypovolaemic), prevention of peri-operative hypothermia is a relevant issue.

Maintenance of body temperature may be helped by the use of insulation (an additional blanket, a space blanket or a warmed-air blanket), by the use of warmed intravenous fluids or by raising the ambient temperature of the operating theatre.

Circulation to the limbs

In long operations, where a patient is kept in one position for a prolonged period (usually several hours), consideration should be given to the circulation to the limbs. The risks are of thromboembolism, ischaemia or even compartment syndrome. It is recommended that the limb in question is either moved or massaged regularly during the operation.

This particularly applies to patients with their legs raised or compressed by the surgical position, for example, patients in Lloyd-Davies stirrups.

Anaesthetic access

The anaesthetist must have easy access to:

- Vascular system (venous and arterial cannulae)
- Airway (e.g. endotracheal tube)
- Monitoring (electrocardiogram (ECG), blood pressure recording, oxygen saturation).

Surgical access

The surgeon should be comfortable during surgery. The operating table should be at the correct height for the surgeon when standing or low enough to allow him to operate sitting down.

The surgical field should be large enough to accommodate the possibility of needing to extend the surgical exposure. This must be borne in mind during patient positioning, skin preparation and draping.

Ancillary theatre equipment

Patient positioning may be influenced by the use of tourniquets, diathermy, image intensifiers, microscopes, endoscopy equipment (such as light sources and monitors) and lasers.

In general, bulky equipment, such as a diathermy machine or an endoscopy monitor, should be positioned on the opposite side to that being operated upon.

When there is a premium on space in the operating theatre, such as when there are a large number of sterile instrument trays as well as a lot of ancillary theatre equipment, it may be helpful to move the operating table away from its usual place in the centre of the operating theatre. For example, a complicated revision right total hip replacement may be performed more easily if the table is moved a short distance to the patient's left.

Use of an image intensifier

When an image intensifier is to be used, its positioning must be borne in mind when positioning the patient. The radiographer should be able to manoeuvre the image intensifier to get clear, uninterrupted imaging of the entire structure that the surgeon needs to visualise. This must be checked after the patient has been positioned and before the skin is prepared and draped.

In some cases, use of the image intensifier must be taken into account before the patient is transferred on to the operating table. If a radiolucent operating table is required, some operating tables are more radiolucent at the foot end of the table. If, say, the humerus needs to be imaged, then it would be necessary to turn the table through 180° so that the patient's head rests at the foot of the table.

As a general rule, the image intensifier receiver, rather than the source, should be on the surgeon's side of the operating table, so that the surgeon receives less radiation exposure.

Theatre staff

During operations involving a surgical approach that is equally visible from either side of the operating table (e.g. a laparotomy or a direct lateral approach to the hip in the lateral position), the scrub nurse should usually stand on the opposite side to the surgeon. Otherwise, the scrub nurse may be able to follow the operation better if standing on the same side as the surgeon.

The surgeon's assistant should generally stand opposite the surgeon. However, if the surgical approach is only visible from one side of the table (e.g. dynamic hip screw fixation of the proximal femur) then the assistant will have to stand next to the surgeon.

Generally the anaesthetist is positioned at the head of the patient, except for head, neck and some shoulder surgery, when access (such as venous access) may be possible only from the foot end. This may involve turning the table round so that the anaesthetic machine is at the foot of the table.

Thromboembolic prophylaxis

Various methods of thromboembolic prophylaxis may be used:

- pharmacological —heparin, low molecular weight heparin (LMWH), warfarin, dextran
- mechanical —early mobilisation, compression stockings, pneumatic compression pumps.

If used, the inflatable boots that form part of a pneumatic compression system will need to be applied in theatre before patient positioning is completed.

Tourniquets

(Figure 12)

Tourniquets are used to create a bloodless surgical field, allowing easier identification of vital structures (such as neurovascular structures).

Application of a tourniquet:

1. Pad the area with soft dressing (e.g. a roll of soft wool padding) to prevent skin wrinkling and blistering under the tourniquet.
2. Apply to the upper arm (Figure 13) or upper thigh (Figure 14) – areas that are well-muscled and afford the major nerves protection from compression.
3. Ensure that the tourniquet is sited proximally enough not to interfere with surgical access when operating at the elbow or knee.
4. Exsanguinate the limb by
   a. using a Rhys-Davies exsanguinator (partly inflated rubber 'sausage'; Figure 15)
   b. applying a compression bandage (rubber Esmarch bandage or crepe bandage)
   c. elevating the limb for 3 to 5 minutes.
   (Partial exsanguination – achieved by elevating the limb for 2 minutes or less – leaves veins partly filled, allowing easier identification of neurovascular bundles.)
5. Inflate to the required pressure. Typical pressures are 250 mmHg in the upper limb and 350 mmHg in the lower limb.
6. Maximum safe tourniquet inflation times: 1.5 hours in the upper limb, 2 hours in the lower limb.
7. Deflate the tourniquet before or after wound closure. The advantages of deflation before closure are:
   a. less peri-operative blood loss as a result of identification (and coagulation) of major bleeding points
   b. less post-operative pain due to a shorter tourniquet inflation time
   c. less patient discomfort if the patient is awake and the tourniquet site is not anaesthetised (e.g. during carpal tunnel release under local anaesthesia).

Note: Be careful not to allow skin preparation fluid to run under the tourniquet. The combination of the fluid and tourniquet pressure can cause a chemical burn. This is a greater risk with alcoholic preparations that are applied prior to tourniquet inflation.

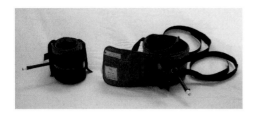

FIG. 12 **Tourniquets**

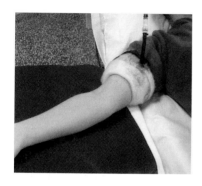

FIG. 13 **High arm tourniquet**

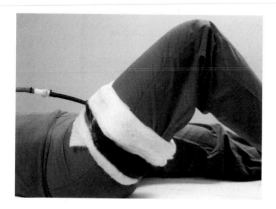

FIG. 14 **Thigh tourniquet, padded and applied with the knee flexed**

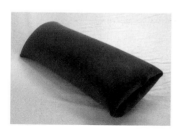

FIG. 15 **Rhys–Davies exsanguinator**

Diathermy

Diathermy injuries are a frequent source of litigation. Knowledge of the safe use of diathermy is mandatory.

What is diathermy?

Diathermy is the passage of an electrical current through tissue, generating heat so as to either coagulate blood vessels (coagulation diathermy) or cut through tissue (cutting diathermy).

Diathermy is a form of electrosurgery.

There are two main types of diathermy circuit:

1. Unipolar diathermy – current passes between the diathermy forceps and a diathermy plate
2. Bipolar diathermy – current passes between the two tips of the diathermy forceps.

Coagulation is produced by a pulsed diathermy output, whereas cutting is produced by a continuous output. 'Blend' allows a combination of both to be used, thus producing greater haemostasis during cutting.

Heating effect

The magnitude of the heating effect of diathermy is related to:

- Current density   —in unipolar diathermy, current density is low at the diathermy plate (large surface area) and high at the tip of the diathermy forceps (small surface area)
- Resistance   —heat is produced where there is resistance to the current flow (usually the tissue at the tip of the diathermy forceps).

Therefore, heat is concentrated at the tip of the diathermy forceps, but it becomes dissipated under the plate, assuming that the plate is applied to an area of the patient that is well vascularised (minimising resistance to current flow).

Unipolar diathermy

The diathermy plate must be applied closely to a well-vascularised area (e.g. thigh, abdomen), as close as practical to the operative field.

Avoid bony prominences or scar tissue, where skin blood flow may be poor.

Consider shaving very hairy patients to allow good contact between the plate and the skin.

It is not good practice to coagulate vessels by touching unipolar diathermy forceps to normal (non-insulated) forceps. Inadvertent adjacent tissue damage may occur.

Bipolar diathermy

Advantage   —safer to use, in that it heats only the tissue between the tips of the diathermy forceps

Disadvantages	—less effective, since less energy can be delivered (unipolar diathermy can deliver up to 10 times more energy) —cannot be used for cutting —will not coagulate when used to touch normal surgical forceps holding a bleeding vessel
Indications	—small operative fields, especially near nerves and near terminal vessels (e.g. hand surgery, penile surgery), where inadvertent coagulation of the vessels may lead to necrosis of the digit or appendage —presence of a cardiac pacemaker.

Diathermy problems

Burns	—incorrect siting of the plate (when using unipolar diathermy) can give rise to a high current density and consequent arcing and skin burns —ignition of spirit used for skin preparation, especially if allowed to pool (may burn with no visible flame) —inadvertent activation of the diathermy forceps whilst they are in contact with tissue away from the operative field —activation of the diathermy forceps whilst they are in contact with a metal object that is touching the patient away from the operative field —inappropriate use of unipolar diathermy within a small operative field, such that delicate tissue adjacent to the target is inadvertently heated (e.g. digital arteries within a finger, leading to ischaemia of the digit)
Pacemakers	—unipolar diathermy may upset cardiac pacemakers, especially if the current crosses the chest and if the pacemaker has been implanted recently
Monitoring	—anaesthetic monitoring (e.g. pulse oximetry, ECG) may be affected by activation of diathermy.

Remember: electrical energy will always take the path of least resistance.

General surgery

Abdomen

Dorsal recumbent position

(Figure 16)

- Supine position on the standard operating table
- Arms by side and tucked in
- Ensure anaesthetist has adequate access
- Padding over elbows to prevent ulnar nerve injury
- One pillow
- When using a head screen avoid contact with the skin and neck
- Ankle supports
- Deep vein thrombosis (DVT) prophylaxis e.g. Anti-embolism stockings or intermittent calf compression
- Warming blanket.

Considerations

- Adequate abdominal exposure. Ensure that exposure above the xiphoid process is obtained especially for upper gastro-intestinal surgery.
- Arm may be abducted to improve venous access.

Surgical approaches

Laparotomy for most abdominal surgery	Laparoscopic surgery, e.g., laparoscopic cholecystectomy, appendicectomy and hernia surgery

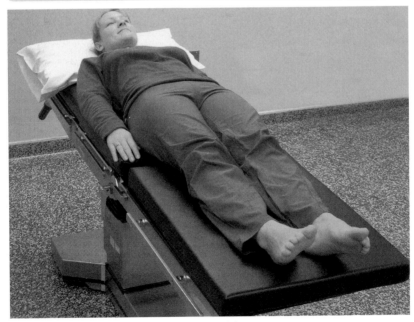

FIG. 16 **Supine (dorsal recumbent) position**

Perineum

Lithotomy position

(Figures 17 and 18)

- Supine position on the operating table
- End of the table removed
- Patient is moved to the lower edge of the operating table with the legs held by an assistant
- The anterior superior iliac spine should be positioned at the level of the break in the table
- The legs are held before being placed in the stirrups
- Legs are usually placed outside of the poles to avoid pressure on the common peroneal nerve.

Considerations

- Avoid hyperflexion of the hips.
- Ensure adequate padding between the legs and poles.
- Avoid overhanging buttocks at the end of the operating table.
- After procedure the feet are returned to the anatomical position in a controlled manner. Pedal pulses are checked and the calves are massaged.

Surgical approaches

Rectum, e.g., abdominal-perineal excision of the rectum

Endoscopic urological procedures

Genitourinary procedure

Perianal procedures

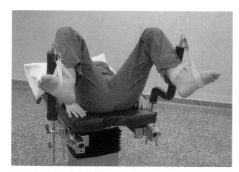

FIG. 17 **Lithotomy position**

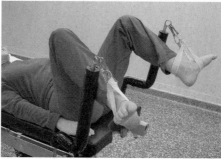

FIG. 18 **Lithotomy position**

Perineum

Lloyd-Davies position

(Figures 19 and 20)

• Similar position as for lithotomy
• Padding especially required around the calves to protect the common peroneal nerve in the lower leg
• The hands can enter the operative field and can also touch the poles. These should be protected by padding and tucked in gently into the body and covered.

Surgical approaches

Rectum especially anterior resection

Genitourinary surgery

Pelvic surgery where access is required from both abdominal and perineal aspects.

Variations

Laparoscopic upper gastrointestinal surgery, e.g., anti-reflux surgery (Figures 21 and 22)

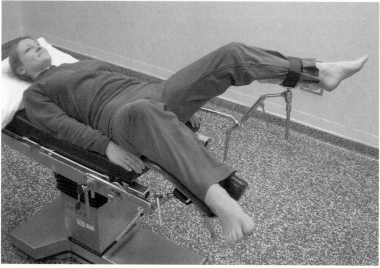

FIG. 19 **Lloyd-Davies position**

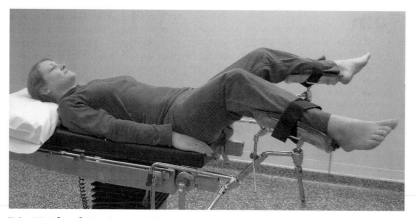

FIG. 20 **Lloyd-Davies position**

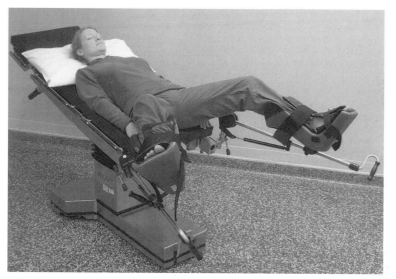

FIG. 21 **Laparoscopic surgery**

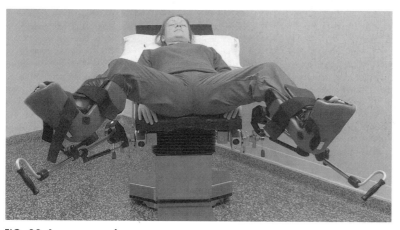

FIG. 22 **Laparoscopic surgery**

Perineum

Jack-knife position

(Figure 23)

- Prone position on the operating table
- The transfer from trolley to the operating table requires team work
- At least four people are required to perform the transfer in addition to the anaesthetist
- Many pillows are required on the operating table to support the body and reduce pressure on the pelvis, back, neck and abdomen
- The head is turned to one side to ensure access to the airway
- The hands and arms can be supported on arm boards
- The extension used for varicose vein surgery can be applied for this purpose and the patient is then placed in the sunbathing position
- The table is then used to achieve the desired position
- Adhesive tape is applied to the patient to keep the surgical position on the operating table and to avoid slipping.

Considerations

- Reduced ventilatory capacity occurs because of compression of the chest and fixity of the abdominal contents.
- Compression of the inferior vena cava from abdominal compression also occurs, which decreases venous return to the heart. This has a cardiovascular effect and also potentially increases the risk of deep vein thrombosis (DVT).
- Transfer from the trolley to table is particularly hazardous because of the possibility of twisting joints especially the arms and hands.

Surgical approaches

Anus

Rectum

Coccyx

Back surgery

Adrenal surgery

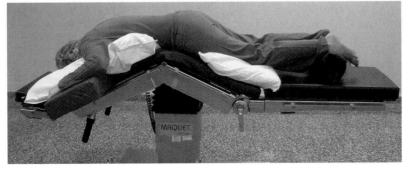

FIG. 23 **Jack-knife position**

Perineum

Knee–chest position

(Figure 24)

- Usual position adopted for sigmoidoscopy without anaesthesia
- Can be lateral or prone
- Patient lies on their side
- Torso lies diagonally across the table
- Hips and knees are flexed
- Avoid straightening at the knees because this may stretch the lumbo-sacral nerves
- Prone position requires the patient to kneel on the table and lower shoulders on to the table so chest and face rest on the table
- Hips and knees in this position remain flexed
- Prone position can be embarrassing for female patients and may be difficult to defend in the presence of adequate alternatives.

Considerations

- Avoid straightening knees as this may injure the lumbo-sacral nerves.
- Prone position more complicated to achieve under general anaesthetic, and it is not advised.

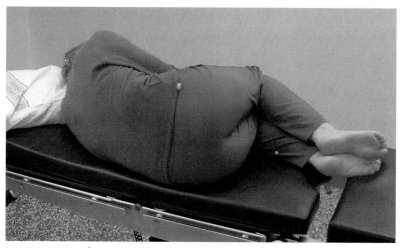

FIG. 24 **Knee–chest position**

Kidney

Lateral kidney position

(Figures 25)

- Patient is anaesthetised in the supine position
- Patient is turned on to their contralateral side, and their back is placed on the edge of the table
- Contralateral kidney placed over the break in the table or over the kidney body elevator if this attachment is available on the table
- The uppermost arm is placed in a gutter rest at no more than 90° abduction or flexion
- Contralateral arm underneath the body is protected with padding
- Contralateral knee is flexed and the uppermost leg is left straight thereby improving the stability of the position
- A large soft pillow is placed between the legs
- Short kidney rest is placed against the back, and a large kidney rest is placed against the abdominal wall with padding
- The entire table is tilted down at the head (Trendelenburg), and the table is broken to curve the body laterally and open up the surgical approach to the kidney
- Kidney strap and tape are placed over the hip to stabilise the patient.

Considerations

- The arms can be a source of problems. Pressure on the contralateral arm underneath the body can cause local effects on nerves, skin or vascular structures.
- The ipsilateral arm, if hyperflexed or abducted, can cause brachial plexus injury.
- Patient may fall off the table at any time until the position is secure.

Surgical approaches

Nephrectomy

Adrenal

Aorta

Lumbar sympathetic trunk

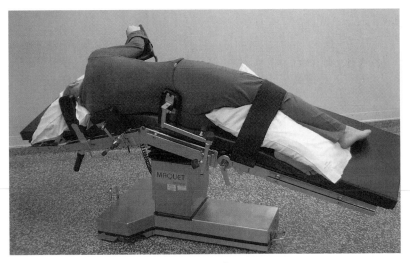

FIG. 25 **Lateral kidney position procedure**

Vascular

Neck and thyroid positions

(Figure 26)

- Patient is placed supine on the operating table
- Neck is placed over the break between the head and thoracic portion of the operating table
- Head extended 10°
- Head placed in a head ring
- A small sandbag may be placed between the shoulders
- A few degrees of negative Trendelenburg tilt (feet down).

Considerations

- The danger of this position is hyperextension of the neck.
- Any neck pathology should be actively excluded by direct questioning prior to the surgery at the preoperative interview.

Surgical approaches

Carotid arterial surgery

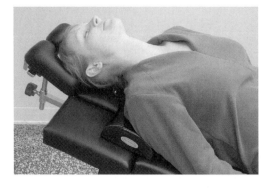

FIG. 26 **Head and neck position**

Vascular

Supine position

(Figure 27)

- Supine position on the standard operating table
- Arms by side and tucked in
- Ensure anaesthetist has adequate access
- Padding over elbows to prevent ulnar nerve injury
- One pillow
- When using a head screen avoid contact with the skin and neck
- Ankle supports
- Deep vein thrombosis (DVT) prophylaxis e.g. TED stockings or intermittent calf compression
- Warming blanket.

> ### Surgical approaches
>
> Aortic aneurysm
>
> Iliac arterial surgery
>
> Axillo-femoral bypass

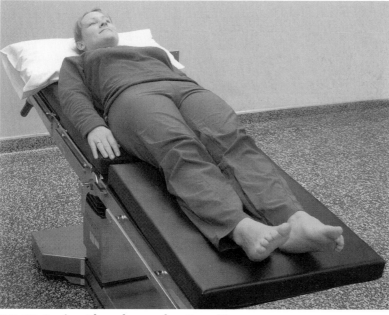

FIG. 27 **Supine (dorsal recumbent) position**

Vascular

Supine position (knee flexed)

(Figure 28)

- Supine position
- Knee flexed
- Hip slightly flexed and externally rotated
- Position is usually obtained by the surgeon after the patient has been prepared and surgically draped.

Considerations

- Surgeon may stand or sit on either side of the distal operative site.
- Hip and knee movements should be performed gently.

Surgical approaches

Femoro-popliteal bypass

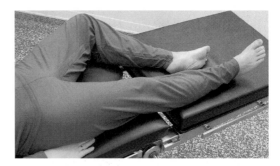

FIG. 28 **Position for femoro-popliteal bypass**

Vascular

Supine position (arm table)

(Figure 29)

- Supine position on a standard operating table
- Attach an arm table to the operating table at the level of the upper chest
- Abduct the arm 60° on to the arm table.

Considerations

- Ensure that any pressure areas are well padded: the occiput, the sacral area, the heels.
- Drape the arm free to allow full shoulder and elbow movement.
- The surgeon usually sits facing the axilla.

> ## Surgical approaches
>
> Forearm arterio-venous fistula

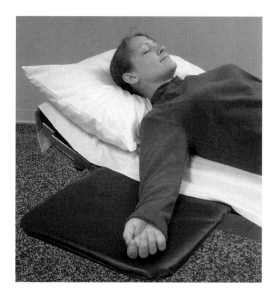

FIG. 29 **Arm abducted on to an arm table, with the arm in neutral (anterior approaches)**

Vascular

Trendelenburg position

(Figure 30)

- Patient is placed in the supine position
- The leg board operating table attachment is placed on the end of the table
- Legs are abducted
- Shoulder braces placed on to the outer parts of the shoulders avoiding the neck
- Body stabilising straps may be applied
- Trendelenburg position with head down performed slowly.

Considerations

- Shoulder braces can cause brachial plexus injury. They should be placed well away from the neck.
- Patient is left in the Trendelenburg position for as short a time as possible.
- Use of a corrugated mattress may reduce risk of slippage.
- Trendelenburg position increases intracerebral pressure and therefore should be avoided if this is of clinical importance.

Surgical approaches

Varicose vein surgery

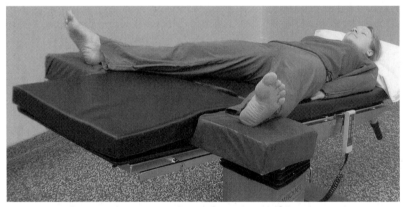

FIG. 30 **Varicose vein surgery (anterior approach)**

Head and neck

Neck and thyroid positions

(Figure 31)

- Patient is placed supine on the operating table
- Neck is placed over the break between the head and thoracic portion of the operating table
- Head extended 10°
- Head placed in a head ring
- A small sandbag may be placed between the shoulders
- A few degrees of negative Trendelenburg tilt (feet down).

Considerations

- The danger of this position is hyperextension of the neck.
- Any neck pathology should be actively excluded by direct questioning prior to the surgery at the preoperative interview.

Surgical approaches

Thyroid

Neck dissection

Parotid gland surgery

Carotid arterial surgery

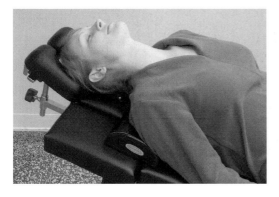

FIG. 31 **Head and neck position**

Breast

Figures 32

- Supine position
- Arm board for axillary dissection.

Considerations

- Avoid hyperabduction of arm of more than 90°.
- Occasionally the arm is draped so that it can be free moving during the surgery or held elevated. In these positions the brachial plexus is vulnerable to injury.
- Breast reconstructive procedures may require the patient to be moved during the procedure for example to procure a latissimus dorsi flap after the excisional surgery has been performed.

Surgical approaches

Breast surgery

Breast reconstruction

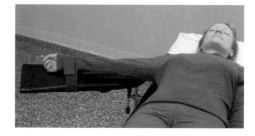

FIG. 32 **Position for breast surgery**

Thorax

Supine position

(Figure 33)

- Supine position on the standard operating table
- Arms by side and tucked in
- Ensure anaesthetist has adequate access
- Padding over elbows to prevent ulnar nerve injury
- One pillow
- When using a head screen avoid contact with the skin and neck
- Ankle supports
- Deep vein thrombosis (DVT) prophylaxis e.g. TED stockings or intermittent calf compression
- Warming blanket.

Surgical approaches

Median sternotomy

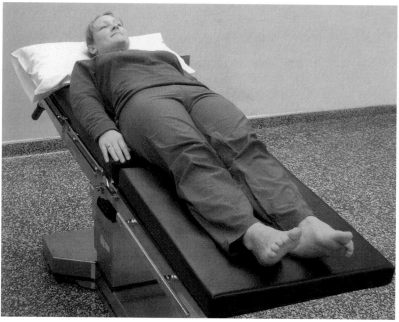

FIG. 33 **Supine (dorsal recumbent) position**

Thorax

Lateral position

(Figure 34)

- The patient is placed on the contralateral side to the operation
- The back is placed on the edge of the table
- The ipsilateral arm is placed in a gutter rest at no more than 90° flexion or 90° abduction
- Contralateral arm is protected by padding under the body
- Contralateral knee is flexed and the uppermost leg is left straight; a soft pillow is placed between the thighs
- A short kidney rest is placed on the back, and a large kidney rest is placed over the abdomen with padding
- Strapping is applied to prevent the patient from slipping.

Considerations

- The arms can be a source of problems. Pressure on the contralateral arm underneath the body can cause local effects on nerves, skin or vascular structures.
- The ipsilateral arm, if hyperflexed or abducted, can cause brachial plexus injury.
- Patient may fall off the table at any time until the position is secure.

Surgical approaches

Lateral thoracotomy

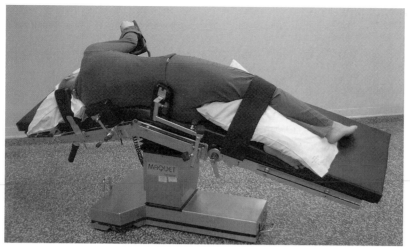

FIG. 34 **Lateral position**

Orthopaedics

Upper limb

Shoulder

Beach-chair position

(Figure 35)

- Supine position on a standard operating table
- Ensure the table break is underneath the lumbosacral area
- Position a support against the lateral chest wall to prevent the patient sliding off the edge of the table (Figure 36)
- The patient should lie as close to the table edge as possible to allow full passive extension of the shoulder – lift the patient against the lumbar support so that the axilla is in line with the edge of the table
- Wedge a small sandbag (or similar support, such as a litre bag of fluid) under the medial border of the scapula to push the shoulder forward
- Elevate the head of the table 30–45° to reduce venous pressure (and thus decrease bleeding) and to allow blood to drain from the operative field
- Laterally flex the neck away from the shoulder, resting the head on a suitable support (e.g. a head ring). Be careful not to flex the neck excessively as this would risk a traction injury to the brachial plexus
- Flex the knees (e.g. over pillows or by breaking the table under the knees) to relieve any tension of the sciatic nerves.

Considerations

- Ensure that any pressure areas are well-padded: the occiput, the areas under the lumbar support, the sacral area, the heels.
- Pad and tape the eyes.
- Drape the arm free to allow full shoulder movement.
- When the head is above the level of the heart, air embolism becomes a potential risk; similarly, cerebral perfusion is reduced, and this may become critical in the presence of hypotension.

Surgical approaches

Anterior (deltopectoral)

Anterolateral (coronal and parasagittal approaches to the acromioclavicular joint)

Lateral (deltoid-splitting)

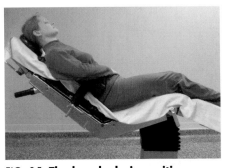

FIG. 35 **The beach-chair position**

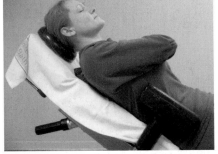

FIG. 36 **The patient is supported by a lateral support placed against the lateral chest wall**

Shoulder

Supine position (intramedullary nailing)

(Figure 37)

- Supine position on a radiolucent operating table
- Wedge a small sandbag (or a litre bag of fluid) under the medial border of the scapula to push the shoulder forward
- Laterally flex the neck away from the shoulder, resting the head on a suitable support (e.g. a pillow or a head ring). Be careful not to flex the neck excessively as this would risk a traction injury to the brachial plexus.

Considerations

- Ensure that any pressure areas are well-padded: the occiput, the sacral area, the heels.
- Drape the arm free to allow full shoulder and elbow movement.
- The image intensifier base may be positioned on the operative side of the table with the C-arm approaching caudally, or it may be positioned on the opposite side of the table with the C-arm passing over the patient. To allow easy access of the C-arm, the patient's head may need to be at the radiolucent leg end of the table (i.e. the table may need to be turned round before the patient is transferred on to it).

Surgical approaches

Antegrade intramedullary nailing of the humerus (via a short lateral deltoid split approach)

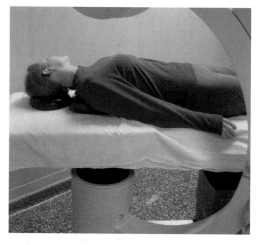

FIG. 37 **Supine position for humeral intramedullary nailing. An image intensifier C-arm is in position for anteroposterior imaging**

Shoulder

Lateral position

(Figure 38)

- Lateral position on a standard operating table (operative side uppermost)
- The patient should lie with their back as close to the table edge as possible
- Position a padded post against the anterior pelvis
- Position a padded lumbar support against the lumbar spine
- Rest the head on a suitable support (e.g. a pillow or a head ring)
- Flex the knees to relieve tension on the sciatic nerves
- Tilt the table into reverse Trendelenburg (head uppermost) to reduce venous pressure (and thus decrease bleeding) and to allow blood to drain from the operative field.

Considerations

- Ensure that the patient is in a stable, well-supported position.
- Ensure that the lower arm is free and not being compressed under the patient's body.
- Support the head sufficiently to keep the neck in a neutral position.
- Ensure that any pressure areas are well-padded: the head, the lower arm, the areas under the post and the lumbar support, the greater trochanter and the lateral malleolus of the lower leg, the medial malleolus of the upper leg.
- Drape the arm free to allow full shoulder movement.
- The surgeon usually stands behind the patient.

Surgical approaches

Anterolateral (coronal and parasagittal approaches to the acromioclavicular joint)

Lateral (deltoid-splitting)

Posterior

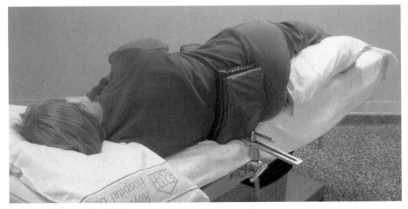

FIG. 38 **Lateral position**

Arm (humerus and elbow)

Prone position

(Figure 39)

- Attach an arm table or a padded gutter (e.g. Carter–Bain) to the operating table at the level of the upper chest
- Transfer the patient on to the operating table in the prone position. This requires rolling the patient from the supine position on to the arms of three or more assistants, who then lift the patient on to the operating table
- In the prone position the patient must have their chest and pelvis supported in order to allow free movement of the abdomen. This may be achieved by lifting the patient on to a special mattress (e.g. the Montreal mattress; see Figure 105)
- Rest the head on a suitable support (e.g. a pillow or a head ring)
- Abduct the contralateral arm 90° and flex the elbow 90° so that the arm lies supported on a suitable arm board
- Abduct the affected arm 90° and place it on the arm table or gutter so that the elbow flexes over the end of the table or gutter, allowing the forearm to hang
- If using an arm table rather than a gutter, consider placing some padding (e.g. a rolled gel pad) under the tourniquet or under the shoulder of the side to be operated on. Alternatively, support the arm on a folded drape after draping.

Considerations

- Ensure that any pressure areas are well-padded: the knees, the pelvis, the external genitalia, the chest, the contralateral arm, the forehead.
- Pad and tape the eyes.
- Move the arms through into position from the side in a front crawl swimming motion (i.e. not simultaneously).
- Flex the knees slightly (e.g. over a pillow) to relieve tension on the sciatic nerves.
- Do not use a tourniquet for operations on the proximal and mid-humerus – it will get in the way.
- Drape the arm free to allow full shoulder and elbow movement.

Surgical approaches

Posterior (humerus and elbow)

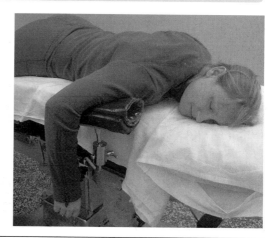

FIG. 39 **Prone position, with the arm abducted over a padded gutter, allowing the forearm to hang**

Arm (humerus and elbow)

Lateral position

(Figures 40 and 41)

- Lateral position on a standard operating table (operative side uppermost)
- The patient should lie centrally on the table so that the upper arm can be positioned easily
- Position a padded post against the anterior pelvis
- Position a padded lumbar support against the lumbar spine
- Rest the head on a suitable support (e.g. a pillow or a head ring)
- Abduct the arm 90° over a padded rest (e.g. a gutter or bar covered with gel padding) so that the elbow can flex, allowing the forearm to hang
- Flex the knees to relieve tension on the sciatic nerves
- Consider tilting the table into reverse Trendelenburg (head uppermost) to reduce venous pressure (and thus decrease bleeding) and to allow blood to drain from the operative field.

Considerations

- Ensure that the patient is in a stable, well-supported position.
- Ensure that the lower arm is free and not being compressed under the patient's body.
- Support the head sufficiently to keep the neck in a neutral position.
- Ensure that no pressure is being applied to the axilla or the antecubital fossa of the elbow.
- Ensure that any pressure areas are well-padded: the head, the lower arm, the areas under the post and the lumbar support, the greater trochanter and the lateral malleolus of the lower leg, the medial malleolus of the upper leg.
- Do not use a tourniquet for operations on the proximal and mid-humerus – it will get in the way.
- Drape the arm free to allow full shoulder and elbow movement.
- The surgeon usually stands behind the patient.

Surgical approaches

Posterior (humerus and elbow)

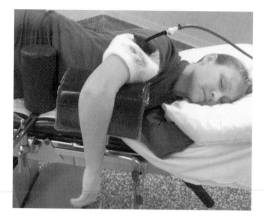

FIG. 40 **Lateral position, with the arm abducted over a padded gutter, allowing the forearm to hang**

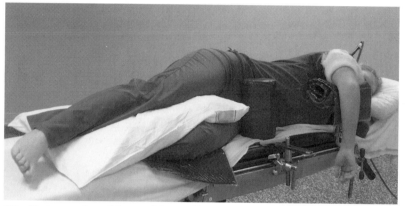

FIG. 41 **Lateral position, with a pillow positioned between the knees**

Arm (humerus and elbow)

Supine position (arm table)

(Figure 42)

- Supine position on a standard operating table
- Attach an arm table to the operating table at the level of the upper chest
- Abduct the arm 60° on to the arm table
- Lateral approaches: internally rotate the arm (or place the arm over the chest – see below)
- Posterolateral approach to the elbow: flex the elbow 90°, internally rotate the arm and pronate the forearm (Figure 43)
- Medial approach to the elbow: externally rotate the arm fully and flex the elbow 90°. Support the forearm (Figure 44).

Considerations

- Ensure that any pressure areas are well-padded: the occiput, the sacral area, the heels.
- A high-arm tourniquet may be used for operations on the distal humerus and elbow (but not for the proximal and mid-humerus – it will only get in the way).
- Drape the arm free to allow full shoulder and elbow movement.
- The surgeon usually sits facing the axilla.

Surgical approaches

Anterior (humerus and elbow)

Anterolateral (Henry approach to humerus and elbow)

Lateral (distal humerus and elbow)

Posterolateral (Kocher approach to elbow/radial head)

Medial (elbow)

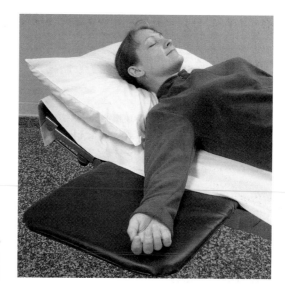

FIG. 42 **Arm abducted on to an arm table, with the arm in neutral (anterior approaches)**

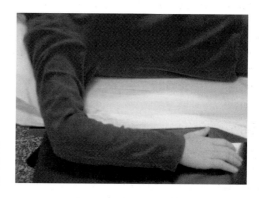

FIG. 43 **Arm internally rotated with the elbow flexed (posterolateral approach)**

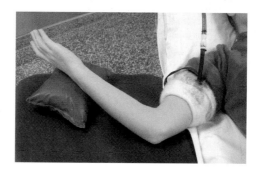

FIG. 44 **Arm externally rotated with the elbow flexed. Note that the forearm is supported**

Arm (humerus and elbow)

Supine position (arm over chest)

(Figure 45)

- Supine position on a standard operating table
- Lie the arm across the patient's chest or abdomen
- Consider tilting the table away from the side to be operated on to help keep the arm in position
- Support the arm on a spare folded drape or on a draped Mayo table (after skin preparation and draping) (Figure 46)
- Posterolateral approach to the elbow: flex the elbow 90° and pronate the forearm
- Posterior approach to the elbow: forward flex the shoulder and support the forearm across the upper chest
- Medial approach to the elbow: to gain adequate exposure this often means flexing the shoulder and elbow so that the forearm lies over the patient's face. This risks affecting the airway and requires an assistant to hold the forearm.

Considerations

- Ensure that any pressure areas are well-padded: the occiput, the sacral area, the heels.
- Remember where the patient is under the drapes and avoid leaning on their face or neck.
- A high-arm tourniquet may be used for operations on the distal humerus and elbow.
- Drape the arm free to allow full shoulder and elbow movement.

Surgical approaches

Lateral (distal humerus and elbow)

Posterolateral (Kocher approach to elbow, radial head)

Posterior (elbow)

Medial (elbow)

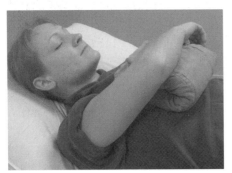

FIG. 45 **Arm placed over the chest with the elbow flexed (posterior approach)**

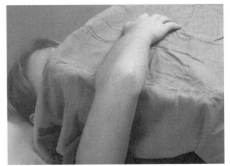

FIG. 46 **Arm placed over a draped Mayo table with the elbow flexed (posterior approach)**

Forearm

Supine position (arm table)

(Figure 47)

- Supine position on a standard operating table
- Attach an arm table to the operating table at the level of the upper chest
- Abduct the arm 60° on to the arm table
- Anterior approach: supinate the forearm
- Posterolateral approach: pronate the forearm (internally rotating the arm and flexing the elbow 90° may also help)
- Medial approach: externally rotate the arm fully and flex the elbow 90°. Support the forearm (Figure 48).

Considerations

- Ensure that any pressure areas are well-padded: the occiput, the sacral area, the heels.
- A high-arm tourniquet is generally used.
- Drape the arm free to allow full shoulder and elbow movement.
- The surgeon usually sits facing the axilla.

Surgical approaches

Anterior (Henry approach to the radius)

Posterolateral (Thompson approach to the radius)

Direct medial (ulna) – elbow flexed

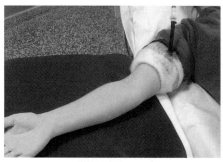

FIG. 47 **Arm abducted on to an arm table, with the forearm supinated (anterior approaches)**

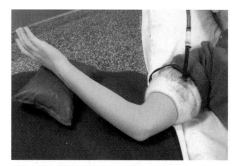

FIG. 48 **Arm externally rotated with the elbow flexed. Note that the forearm is supported**

Forearm

Supine position (arm over chest)

(Figure 49)

- Supine position on a standard operating table
- Lie the arm across the patient's chest
- Consider tilting the table away from the side to be operated on to help keep the arm in position
- Support the arm on a spare folded drape or on a draped Mayo table (after skin preparation and draping)
- Posterolateral approach to the radius: supinate the forearm (or keep it in neutral)
- Direct medial approach: pronate the forearm.

Considerations

- Ensure that any pressure areas are well-padded: the occiput, the sacral area, the heels.
- Remember where the patient is under the drapes and avoid leaning on their face or neck.
- A high-arm tourniquet may be used for operations on the distal humerus and elbow.
- Drape the arm free to allow full shoulder and elbow movement.

Surgical approaches

Posterolateral (Thompson approach to the radius)

Direct medial (ulna)

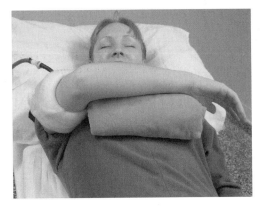

FIG. 49 **Arm placed over the chest with the elbow flexed and forearm pronated (medial approach)**

Wrist and hand

Supine position (arm table)

(Figures 50 and 51)

- Supine position on a standard operating table
- Attach an arm table to the operating table at the level of the upper chest
- Abduct the arm 60° on to the arm table
- Dorsal approaches: pronate the forearm (so that the palm faces downwards)
- Volar approaches: supinate the forearm (so that the palm faces upwards).

Considerations

- Ensure that any pressure areas are well-padded: the occiput, the sacral area, the heels.
- A high-arm tourniquet is generally used.
- Drape the arm free to allow full shoulder and elbow movement.
- The surgeon usually sits facing the axilla.

Surgical approaches

Dorsal (posterior) approaches

Volar (palmar/anterior) approaches

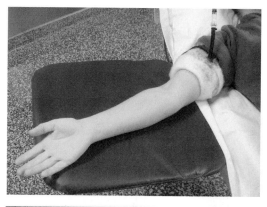

FIG. 50 **Arm abducted on to an arm table, with the forearm supinated (anterior approaches)**

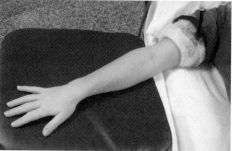

FIG. 51 **Arm abducted on to an arm table, with the forearm pronated (dorsal approaches)**

Lower limb

Pelvis

Supine position

(Figure 52)

- Supine position on a standard operating table
- Place a small sandbag (or a similar support) under the buttock of the side to be operated on. This will elevate the iliac crest and rotate it internally, thus improving access
- Anterior approach to sacroiliac joint: position a lumbar support against the opposite iliac wing and tilt the table 20° away, so that the pelvic contents fall away (Figure 53).

Considerations

- Ensure that any pressure areas are well-padded: the occiput, the sacral area, the heels.

Surgical approaches

Anterior approach to the iliac crest

Anterior approach to the pubic symphysis

Anterior approach to the sacroiliac joint

Alternative

Posterior approaches (to the iliac crest and the sacroiliac joint) may be performed with the patient in a prone position (see Lumbar spine).

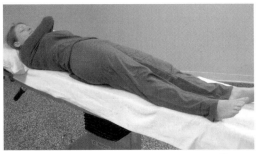

FIG. 52 **Supine position. Note the sandbag under the buttock, raising the hip forward**

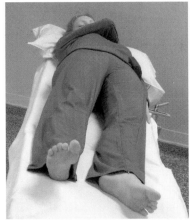

FIG. 53 **Supine position. The table has been tilted 20° away from the operated side, the patient being supported by a support against the opposite iliac wing**

Hip

Supine position (medial approach)

(Figure 54)

- Supine position on a standard operating table
- The hip to be operated on should be flexed, abducted and externally rotated, so that the foot lies along the medial side of the contralateral knee.

Considerations

- Ensure that any pressure areas are well-padded: the occiput, the sacral area, the heels.
- Drape the leg free to allow full hip and knee movement.

Surgical approaches

Medial (Ludloff) approach to the hip

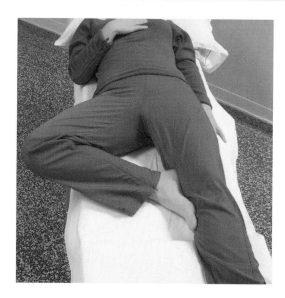

FIG. 54 **Supine position with the hip flexed, abducted and externally rotated (medial approach to the hip)**

Hip

Supine position (anterior and lateral approaches)

(Figure 55)

- Supine position on a standard operating table
- Place a small sandbag (or a similar support) under the buttock of the side to be operated on. This will raise the hip forward and will help improve access
- Anterolateral and direct lateral approaches to the hip (and the ilioinguinal approach to the acetabulum): position the patient close to the edge of the table so that the buttock hangs over the edge, and also tilt the table 20° away. Both manoeuvres allow the gluteal fat and gluteal muscles to fall away from the operative field.

Considerations

- Ensure that any pressure areas are well-padded: the occiput, the sacral area, the heels.
- Pelvic surgery: insert a urethral catheter to empty the bladder.
- Drape the leg free to allow full hip and knee movement.

Surgical approaches

Ilioinguinal approach to the acetabulum

Anterior (iliofemoral or Smith-Petersen) approach to the hip

Anterior (extended iliofemoral) approach to the acetabulum

Anterolateral (Watson-Jones) approach to the hip

Direct lateral (transgluteal or Hardinge) approach to the hip

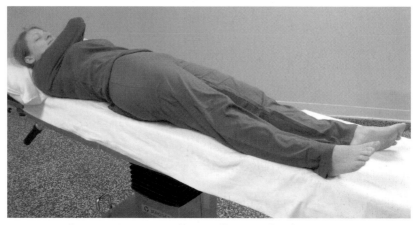

FIG. 55 **Supine position. Note the sandbag under the buttock, raising the hip forward**

Hip

Lateral position

(Figure 56)

- True lateral position on a standard operating table (operative side uppermost)
- Position a padded post against the anterior pelvis (the anterior superior iliac spines)
- Position a padded lumbar support against the lumbar spine
- Rest the head on a suitable support (e.g. a pillow or a head ring)
- Flex the knees to relieve tension of the sciatic nerves.

Considerations

- Ensure that the patient is in a stable, well-supported position.
- Ensure that the lower arm is free and not being compressed under the patient's body.
- Support the head sufficiently to keep the neck in a neutral position.
- Ensure that any pressure areas are well-padded: the head, the lower arm, the areas under the post and the lumbar support, the greater trochanter and the lateral malleolus of the lower leg, the medial malleolus of the upper leg.
- Place a pillow between the knees (Figure 57).
- Check that the leg can be moved sufficiently to allow full access to the medullary canal of the femur.
- Drape the leg free to allow full hip and knee movement.
- The surgeon usually stands behind the patient during surgery.

Surgical approaches

Direct lateral (Hardinge or transgluteal) approach to the hip

Posterior (Moore or southern) approach to the hip

Posterior approach to the acetabulum

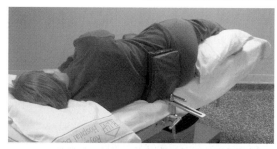

FIG. 56 **Lateral position**

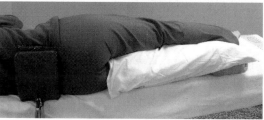

FIG. 57 **Lateral position**

Thigh (femur)

Supine position (with traction)

(Figure 58)

- Supine position on an orthopaedic traction table, with leg extension supports replacing the conventional foot end of the table (see Figure 9)
- Place a well-padded perineal post into the appropriate hole in the table for counter-traction. The correct hole is usually to the same side as the leg to be operated on. Inserting the post may require abducting the leg or even lifting the patient up the table temporarily
- In conjunction with the anaesthetist looking after the head and neck of the patient, lift the patient down against the perineal post, such that traction will be applied against the ipsilateral pubic rami (not against the external genitalia)
- The ipsilateral arm should be secured across the patient's chest
- Move each leg into position and secure it to the traction attachment. The configuration of the traction attachment will vary according to the desired method of applying traction (see below)
- Remove each leg extension support
- Adjust the position of the leg to be operated on and apply traction as required. As a precaution, support the leg with your hand as traction is applied
- Check that the image intensifier can image the entire surgical area (posteroanterior and lateral views) and check the reduction of any fracture.

Configuration of the traction attachment:

- Methods of applying traction:
  - Traction boot (Figure 59). After padding the foot (e.g. using a roll of soft wool padding) secure the foot within the traction boot. Make sure that the heel is seated fully into the boot and that the straps are tightened firmly. For added security, especially if traction is to be applied, firmly wrap a bandage around the boot and lower leg of the patient in a figure-of-8 fashion (Figure 60). Then attach the boot to a vertical traction bar attached to a traction arm.
    If traction needs to be applied to a leg that has previously been amputated below-knee, then it may be possible to place the below-knee amputation stump into an inverted traction boot (Figure 61)
  - Traction pin. A distal femoral (transcondylar) (Figure 62) or a proximal tibial traction pin (Figure 63) is inserted and then attached to a traction stirrup. The stirrup is then secured to a vertical traction bar attached to either a traction arm or central traction bar
- Position of the contralateral leg. This determines whether the traction table is set up using a pair of traction arms or a central traction bar:
  1. Flex and abduct the leg, after securing the padded foot within a traction boot, and then attach the boot to one of the traction arms (see Figure 58)
  2. Drop the leg into extension, after securing the padded foot within a traction boot, and then attach the boot to one of the traction arms (see Figure 65)
  3. Drop the leg into extension and rest the calf in a gutter attached to the central traction bar (see Figure 64). The gutter should be lined with gel padding and the leg should be firmly bandaged in place.

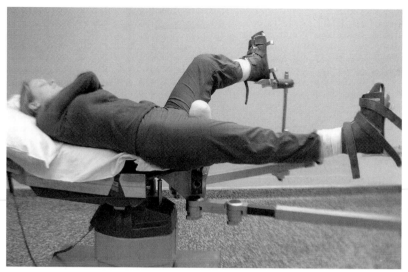

FIG. 58 **The DHS position. Traction is applied via a traction boot, with the ipsilateral leg in neutral or slight internal rotation and the contralateral leg flexed and abducted**

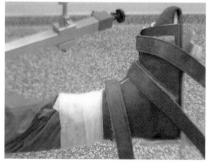

FIG. 59 **Traction boot. Note that the foot has been padded**

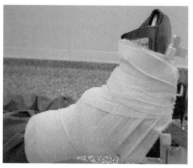

FIG. 60 **The foot is kept securely within the traction boot using firm bandaging**

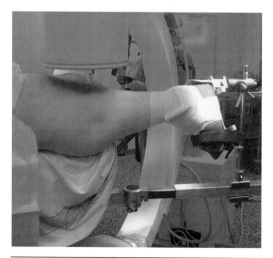

FIG. 61 **Traction being applied to the leg of a below-knee amputee. The stump has been fixed into an inverted traction boot**

The leg must be positioned so as to allow a clear, unhindered imaging of the leg to be operated on.

Internal fixation of the proximal femur (dynamic hip screw fixation or cannulated screw fixation) (see Figure 58):

- Traction arms should be used, both with vertical traction bars attached
- Pad both feet and secure them within traction boots. The ipsilateral foot should be additionally held by firmly bandaging the boot and lower leg in a figure-of-8 fashion
- Ipsilateral leg. With the leg aligned in neutral (hip in neutral and knee extended), attach the boot to the vertical traction bar. Internally rotate the leg 15° to overcome the natural anteversion of the femoral neck and thus bring the lateral cortex of the proximal femur into a true lateral position. Check that the leg is horizontal (parallel to the floor)
- Contralateral leg: gently flex and abduct the leg, before attaching the boot to the vertical traction bar. Check that image intensifier can be manoeuvred easily to provide posteroanterior and oblique lateral views of the proximal femur
- Apply traction as required and check the reduction of any fracture. A satisfactory closed reduction of most proximal femoral fractures may be achieved just by applying traction in the position described.

Intramedullary nailing of the femur (Figures 64 and 65):

- Traction arms or a central traction bar may be used, according to whether the contralateral leg is to be placed in a boot or a gutter
- Adduct (laterally flex) the trunk away from the operative side to allow unobstructed passage of the intramedullary guidewire, reamers and nail
- Consider placing a pillow (or similar support) under the lumbar spine to increase the patient's lumbar lordosis, which may improve access
- Ipsilateral leg. The leg may be secured either by placing the foot within a traction boot (Figure 65) or by inserting a traction pin and attaching this to a traction stirrup (Figure 64). Attach the boot or stirrup to a vertical traction bar. The leg should initially be horizontal or in slight (15–30°) flexion and in neutral rotation (toes pointing upwards if a boot is used or tibia hanging vertically downwards if a traction pin is used)
- Contralateral leg. For standard femoral nailing, where the proximal locking screws pass across the intertrochanteric area, the contralateral leg may be dropped into extension for the duration of the surgery. Lateral views of the proximal femur will need to be slightly oblique, but this will usually prove to be satisfactory. Dropping the contralateral leg into extension allows an unimpeded horizontal beam lateral image of the distal femur to be taken, which is essential for easy distal locking. For femoral nailing involving the insertion of proximal locking devices up the femoral neck (e.g. reconstruction femoral nailing), the contralateral leg should be flexed and abducted for proximal locking (see Figure 58) and then dropped into extension for distal locking. It is important to get a good quality lateral image of the femoral neck during proximal locking
- Adjust the position of the leg to be operated on and apply traction as required to achieve an adequate reduction. As a precaution, support the leg with your hand as traction is applied

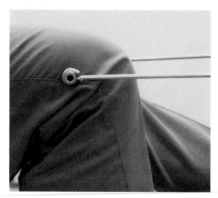

FIG. 62 **Distal femoral (transcondylar) traction**

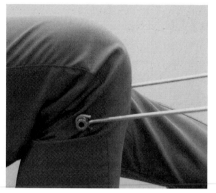

FIG. 63 **Proximal tibial traction**

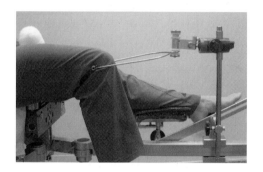

FIG. 64 **Traction set-up for femoral intramedullary nailing. Traction is applied via a distal femoral traction pin and traction stirrup. The contralateral leg is resting in a padded gutter**

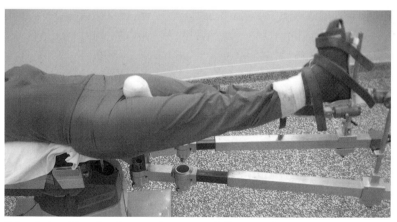

FIG. 65 **Position for femoral intramedullary nailing. Traction is applied via a traction boot, with the ipsilateral leg slightly flexed and the contralateral leg extended**

- Proximal fractures: adduct the trunk away from the operative side and keep the leg in neutral
- Distal fractures: keep the trunk in neutral, adduct the leg and consider extending the knee. If the hip is arthritic it may be necessary to flex the hip to allow sufficient adduction
- Check that the entire femur can be imaged satisfactorily.

Internal fixation of the femoral shaft and distal femur:

- Traction arms or a central traction bar may be used, according to whether the contralateral leg is to be placed in a boot or a gutter
- Ipsilateral leg. The leg may be secured either by placing the foot within a traction boot or by inserting a traction pin and attaching this to a traction stirrup. Attach the boot or stirrup to a vertical traction bar. The leg should initially be horizontal and in neutral rotation (toes pointing upwards if a boot is used or tibia hanging vertically downwards if a traction pin is used)
- Contralateral leg. An unimpeded horizontal beam lateral image of the femoral shaft or distal femur is best achieved by dropping the contralateral leg into extension.
- Apply traction as required and check the reduction of any fracture. Adjust the position of the leg as necessary to improve the reduction.

Considerations

- Ensure that any pressure areas are well-padded: the occiput, the sacral area, the perineum, the contralateral calf (if in a gutter), the heels (within traction boots).
- Ensure that there is no compression of the external genitalia.
- When placing a patient into position on traction, always hold the patient's leg and move it into position before securing it to the traction extension. Moving the leg after it has been secured to the extension applies considerable leverage to the leg, which may result in an iatrogenic fracture, especially in elderly patients with osteoporotic bones.
- If a ligamentous injury of the knee is suspected, traction should be applied via a distal femoral traction pin, rather than via a proximal tibial pin or a traction boot. Not only will applying traction across the knee aggravate the ligamentous injury but, in the absence of adequate ligamentous restraints, the neurovascular structures may be stretched with disastrous consequences.
- If using a traction boot, be aware that patients with small feet can slide out of the boot when traction is applied.
- The image intensifier base should be positioned on the opposite side of the table with the C-arm passing over the patient. To allow easy access of the C-arm the patient's head may need to be at the foot end of the table (i.e. the table may need to be turned round before the patient is transferred on to it).

Surgical approaches

Lateral – allows access to entire femur from trochanteric area (e.g. dynamic hip screw fixation) to femoral shaft (plating) to distal femur (e.g. dynamic condylar screw fixation).

Thigh (femur)

Supine position (without traction)

(Figure 66)

- Supine position on a radiolucent operating table
- Check that the image intensifier can image the entire surgical area (anteroposterior and lateral views)
- Lateral approach to proximal femur: an adequate lateral view of the femoral neck (e.g. for cannulated screw fixation of a slipped upper femoral epiphysis) may be obtained by keeping the C-arm of the image intensifier vertical and flexing, abducting and externally rotating the hip, so that the foot lies along the medial side of the contralateral knee (similar to the position for a medial approach to the hip (see above)
- Posterolateral approach to the femur: place a small sandbag (or a similar support) under the buttock of the side to be operated on. This will raise the hip forward and will help improve access.

Considerations

- Ensure that any pressure areas are well-padded: the occiput, the sacral area, the heels.
- The image intensifier base should be positioned on the opposite side of the table with the C-arm passing over the patient.
- Drape the leg free to allow full hip and knee movement.

Surgical approaches

Lateral

Anteromedial (distal two thirds of femur)

Posterolateral

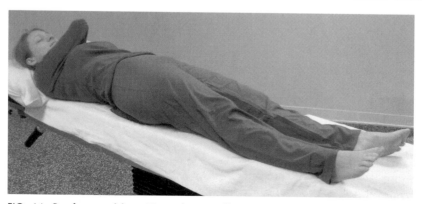

FIG. 66 **Supine position. Note the sandbag under the buttock, raising the hip forward**

Thigh (femur)

Lateral position (with traction)

(Figures 67 and 68)

- The orthopaedic traction table, with leg extension supports replacing the conventional foot end of the table, should be set up with vertical traction bars attached to the traction arms
- Transfer the patient on to the table supine
- To apply traction to the ipsilateral leg, the foot may be placed into a traction boot or a distal femoral or proximal tibial traction pin may be inserted. If a boot is used the foot must be padded and the boot and lower leg should be bandaged firmly in figure-of-8 fashion
- The foot of the contralateral leg should be padded and secured within a traction boot
- Turn the patient into a true lateral position (operative side uppermost)
- Abduct the upper leg and insert a well-padded horizontal perineal post between the legs
- With the anaesthetist looking after the head and neck of the patient, lift the patient down against the perineal post, which should be adjusted so that traction will be applied against the ipsilateral pubic rami (not against the external genitalia)
- Position a padded post against the anterior chest wall
- Position a padded lumbar support against the thoracic spine
- Rest the head on a suitable support (e.g. a pillow or a head ring)
- Attach each leg to its vertical traction bar, via either a traction boot or a traction pin attached to a traction stirrup
  - Ipsilateral leg. Flex the hip 15–30° and keep the knee extended. Internally rotate the leg 15° to overcome the natural anteversion of the femoral neck and thus bring the lateral cortex of the proximal femur into a true lateral position. Check that the leg is horizontal (parallel to the floor)
  - Contralateral leg. Keep the leg in neutral or slight hip flexion
- Check that the image intensifier can be manoeuvred easily to provide satisfactory posteroanterior and vertical beam lateral views of the entire femur. The C-arm may need to be slightly oblique to obtain a lateral view of the femoral neck
- Apply traction, supporting the leg with your hand as traction is applied. Adduction of the fractured femur may be required to achieve an adequate reduction and allow unobstructed passage of the guidewire, reamers and nail. If the hip is arthritic it may be necessary to flex the hip further to allow sufficient adduction
- Use of the lateral position for intramedullary nailing is particularly useful if the patient is obese.

Considerations

- Ensure that the patient is in a stable, well-supported position.
- Ensure that the lower arm is free and not being compressed under the patient's body.
- Support the head sufficiently to keep the neck in a neutral position.
- Ensure that any pressure areas are well-padded: the head, the areas under the anterior post and the lumbar support, the lower arm, the perineum, the heels (within traction boots).

- Ensure that there is no compression of the external genitalia.
- Place a pillow between the knees.
- Drape the leg free to allow full hip and knee movement.
- The surgeon usually stands behind the patient during surgery.

Surgical approaches

Lateral (intramedullary nailing of the femur)

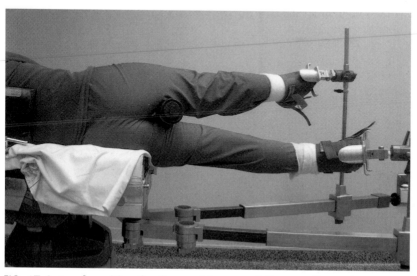

FIG. 67 **Lateral position for femoral intramedullary nailing. The ipsilateral hip is flexed 15–30°. A horizontal perineal post is used for counter-traction**

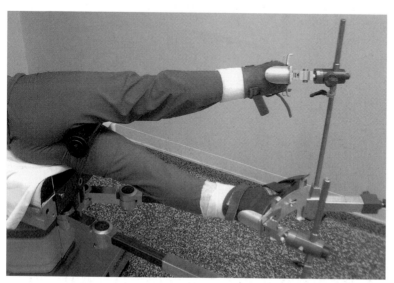

FIG. 68 **Lateral position for femoral intramedullary nailing. The ipsilateral hip is flexed 15–30°. A horizontal perineal post is used for counter-traction**

Thigh (femur)

Lateral position (without traction)

(Figure 69)

- True lateral position on a standard operating table (operative side uppermost)
- Position a padded post against the anterior pelvis
- Position a padded lumbar support against the lumbar spine
- Rest the head on a suitable support (e.g. a pillow or a head ring)
- Flex the knees to relieve tension of the sciatic nerves.

Considerations

- Ensure that the patient is in a stable, well-supported position.
- Ensure that the lower arm is free and not being compressed under the patient's body.
- Ensure that any pressure areas are well-padded: the areas under the post and the lumbar support, the greater trochanter and the lateral malleolus of the lower leg, the medial malleolus of the upper leg.
- Place a pillow between the knees.
- Drape the leg free to allow full hip and knee movement.
- The surgeon usually stands behind the patient during surgery.

> ### Surgical approaches
> Lateral
>
> #### Alternative
> A posterior approach to the femur may be performed with the patient in a prone position (see Lumbar spine).

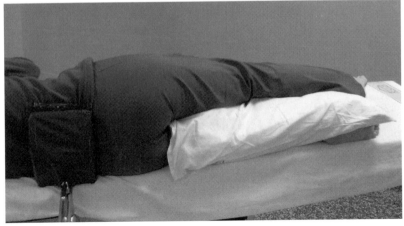

FIG. 69 **Lateral position**

Knee

Supine position (anterior and lateral approaches)

(Figure 70)

- Supine position on a standard operating table
- If a thigh tourniquet is to be used, apply the tourniquet as high as possible. This is most easily achieved with the hip flexed and abducted and the knee flexed. Inflate the tourniquet with the knee flexed (so that the quadriceps muscle is not 'tethered' by the tourniquet)
- A suitable support (such as a sandbag taped to the table or a horizontal cylindrical support (see Figure 7) may be used to keep the knee flexed by preventing the foot from sliding. The knee may either be supported in 90° flexion (the optimal position for opening and closing an anterior midline approach) or in maximum flexion (the main operating position during a total knee replacement) (Figure 71). If the latter position is used, the knee may be temporarily supported in 45° flexion for wound opening and closure by placing a few folded drapes beneath the knee (Figure 72)
- To prevent the knee flopping laterally when flexed, a support can be positioned against the upper thigh, so that the tibia is held vertically (Figure 73).

Alternative (Figure 74)

- Supine position on a standard operating table, with the knee positioned over the junction between the middle section and the end (foot) section of the table
- Place a sandbag or similar beneath the distal thigh (but not so that the popliteal fossa is compressed)
- Remove or drop the end of the table ('break' the table) to allow the knee to flex at least 90° over the end of the table.

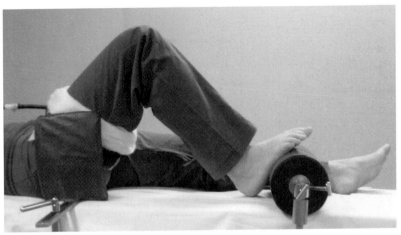

FIG. 70 **Knee supported in 90° flexion using a horizontal foot support. A side support against the tourniquet prevents the knee from falling outwards**

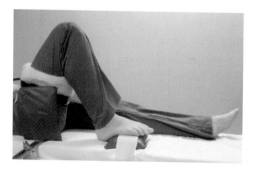

FIG. 71 **Knee supported in 90°
flexion using a sandbag taped to
the table**

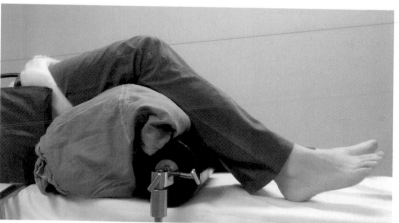

FIG. 72 **Knee supported in semi-flexion using folded drapes under
the knee**

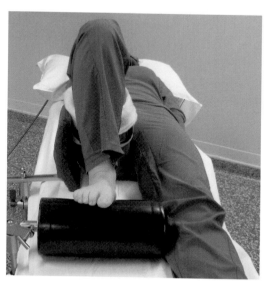

FIG. 73 **A side support
prevents the flexed knee from
falling outwards**

Considerations

- Ensure that any pressure areas are well-padded: the occiput, the sacral area, the heels.
- If a tourniquet is used, beware of trapping the genitalia under the tourniquet.
- Drape the leg free to allow full hip and knee movement.
- For anterior approaches the surgeon may stand on either side of the table. For example, right-handed surgeons may find it easier to operate on a left knee from the contralateral side. Alternatively, the surgeon may sit at the end of the table if the knee is flexed over the end of a 'broken' table.

Surgical approaches

Anterior (medial or lateral parapatellar)

Lateral

Cruciate ligament reconstruction (open or arthroscopic)

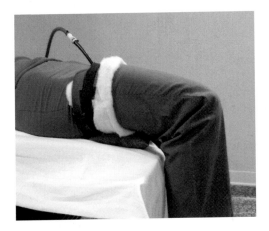

FIG. 74 **Knee flexed over the end of the table, with a sandbag under the thigh tourniquet**

Knee

Supine position (medial approach)

(Figure 75)

- Supine position on a standard operating table
- Flex the knee to be operated on about 60° and abduct and externally rotate the hip, so that the foot lies across the contralateral leg (shin) – this is commonly referred to as the 'figure-of-4' position.

Considerations

- Ensure that any pressure areas are well-padded: the occiput, the sacral area, the heels.
- A thigh tourniquet may be used for operations on the knee.
- Drape the leg free to allow full hip and knee movement.

Surgical approaches

Medial approach

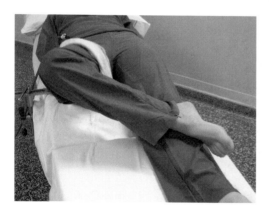

FIG. 75 **Figure-of-4 position for knee arthroscopy (lateral compartment)**

Knee

Supine position (arthroscopy)

(Figures 76 and 77)

- Supine position on a standard operating table
- To view the medial compartment a valgus force needs to be applied to the knee. This is made easier if some form of support is positioned to stop the thigh moving laterally. This is commonly either a lumbar support positioned level with the lateral aspect of the upper thigh (or the thigh tourniquet) (Figure 76) or a specialised leg holder into which the thigh is clamped (Figure 78). The thigh should be allowed to move laterally enough to allow the foot to move off the table so that the knee can be flexed easily
- To view the lateral compartment, flex the knee and abduct and externally rotate the hip into the 'figure-of-4' position (Figure 77).

Considerations

- Ensure pressure areas are well-padded: areas under post and lumbar support, greater trochanter and lateral malleolus of lower leg, medial malleolus of upper leg.
- A thigh tourniquet is commonly used.
- Drape the leg free to allow full shoulder movement.

Surgical approaches

Medial compartment (valgus force using a leg holder or side support)

Lateral compartment (figure-of-4 position)

Alternative

A posterior approach to the femur may be performed with the patient in a prone position (see Lumbar spine).

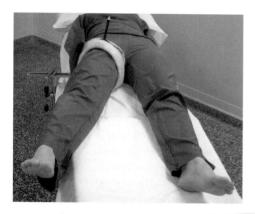

FIG. 76 **Valgus position for knee arthroscopy (medial compartment)**

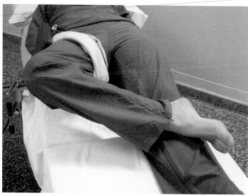

FIG. 77 **Figure-of-4 position for knee arthroscopy (lateral compartment)**

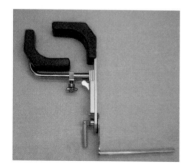

FIG. 78 **Arthroscopic leg holder. The thigh tourniquet is placed within the thigh clamp**

Leg (tibia and fibula)

Supine position (with traction)

(Figure 79)

- Supine position on an orthopaedic traction table, with leg extension supports replacing the conventional foot end of the table (see Figure 9)
- Insert a vertical bar between the patient's legs into an appropriate hole in the table. The patient may need to be lifted up the table temporarily to achieve this. The correct hole is usually to the same side as the leg to be operated on. Attach a well-padded horizontal cylindrical post to the vertical bar (Figure 80) and then lift the leg over the post
- In conjunction with the anaesthetist looking after the head and neck of the patient, lift the patient down against the horizontal post so that the post supports the distal thigh of the ipsilateral leg and the hip is flexed to approximately 70–90°. Do not allow the post to press into the popliteal fossa, where it may cause nerve injury. Side supports may need to be placed against the femoral condyles to stop the knee flopping sideways
- Move each leg into position and secure it to the traction attachment. The configuration of the traction attachment will vary according to the desired method of applying traction (see below)
- Remove each leg extension support
- Adjust the position of the leg to be operated on and apply traction as required. As a precaution, support the leg with your hand as traction is applied
- The ipsilateral tibia should be horizontal to facilitate manipulation of the image intensifier C-arm
- Rotational alignment is achieved by aligning the iliac crest, patella and second ray of the foot
- Check that the image intensifier can image the entire surgical area (posteroanterior and lateral views) and check the reduction of any fracture.

Configuration of the traction attachment:

- Methods of applying traction:
  - Traction boot (see Figure 59). After padding the foot (e.g. using a roll of soft wool padding) secure the foot within the traction boot. Make sure that the heel is seated fully into the boot and that the straps are tightened firmly. For added security, especially if traction is to be applied, firmly wrap a bandage around the boot and lower leg of the patient in a figure-of-8 fashion. Then attach the boot to a vertical traction bar attached to a traction arm
  - Foot holder. A boot is usually inappropriate as the boot will cover the distal tibia and, for example, will prevent distal locking of an intramedullary tibial nail. However, it may be possible to secure the foot to a foot holder. If a specialised foot holder is not available, a foot holder can be manufactured by removing a traction boot from its foot-plate, padding the plate with a gel pad and then firmly strapping the foot to the padded foot-plate (Figure 81). The strapping should not extend above the ankle or otherwise it will interfere with distal locking
  - Traction pin (see Figure 79). A calcaneal skeletal traction pin is inserted and

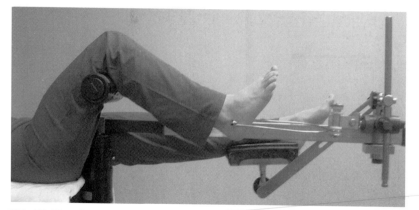

FIG. 79 **Traction set-up for tibial intramedullary nailing. Traction is applied via a calcaneal traction pin and traction stirrup, with counter-traction provided by a horizontal distal thigh support. The contralateral leg is resting in a padded gutter**

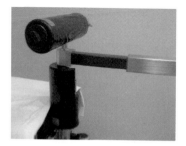

FIG. 80 **Traction attachment for tibial intramedullary nailing, consisting of a padded perineal post, a horizontal thigh support and a central traction bar**

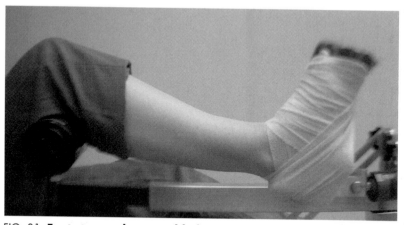

FIG. 81 **Foot strapped to a padded traction foot-plate with firm bandaging**

then attached to a traction stirrup. The stirrup is then secured to a vertical traction bar attached to either a traction arm or central traction bar
- Position of the contralateral leg. This determines whether the traction table is set up using a pair of traction arms or a central traction bar:
  1. Flex and abduct the leg, after securing the padded foot within a traction boot, and then attach the boot to one of the traction arms
  2. Drop the leg into extension, after securing the padded foot within a traction boot, and then attach the boot to one of the traction arms
  3. Drop the leg into extension and rest the calf in a gutter attached to the central traction bar. The gutter should be lined with gel padding and the leg should be firmly bandaged in place.

The leg must be positioned so as to allow a clear, unhindered imaging of the leg to be operated on.

Theatre set-up

There are essentially two basic configurations (Figures 82 and 83):

1. Conventionally, the surgeon performs the majority of the surgery from the lateral side (the ipsilateral side of the table). As distal locking is most safely performed from the medial side the surgeon needs to change sides to perform distal locking

   The image intensifier base should be positioned on the opposite contralateral side of the table with the C-arm passing over the patient. The receiver, rather than the source, should be on the surgeon's side when a horizontal beam lateral image is being taken
2. A more efficient method, which is also less likely to result in wound contamination, is to perform all the surgery from the medial side

   The surgeon, scrub nurse and assistant all stand on the medial side. The surgeon may need to stand on a foot platform

   The image intensifier base should be positioned on the ipsilateral side of the table. The receiver, rather than the source, should be on the surgeon's side when a horizontal beam lateral image is being taken.

Considerations

- Ensure that any pressure areas are well-padded: the occiput, the sacral area, the perineum, the popliteal fossa of the ipsilateral knee, the calf of the contralateral leg (if in a gutter), the heels (if within traction boots or strapped to a foot-plate).
- When placing a patient into position on traction, always hold the patient's leg and move it into position before securing it to the traction extension. Moving the leg after it has been secured to the extension applies considerable leverage to the leg, which may result in an iatrogenic fracture, especially in elderly patients with osteoporotic bones.
- Do not use a tourniquet.

Surgical approaches

Anterior

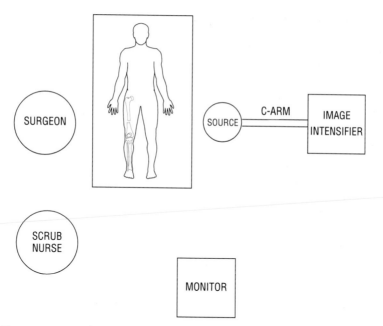

FIG. 82 **Theatre set-up for tibial intramedullary nailing – surgeon standing laterally**

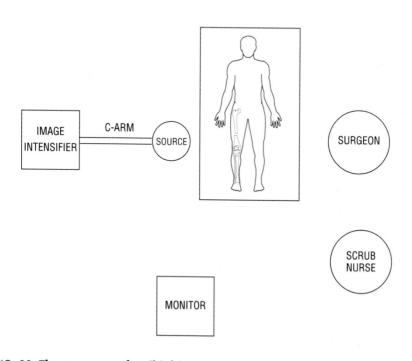

FIG. 83 **Theatre set-up for tibial intramedullary nailing – surgeon standing medially**

Leg (tibia and fibula)

Supine position (without traction)

- Supine position on a standard operating table (may need to be radiolucent)
- Anteromedial approach: the leg naturally lies in slight external rotation when a patient is supine (see Figure 86). To increase external rotation, the figure-of-4 position may be used (see above)
- Anterolateral and posterolateral approaches: place a sandbag under the buttock to help internally rotate the leg (see Figure 87)
- Intramedullary nailing (without traction = freehand). The table must be radiolucent. Check that the image intensifier can image the entire tibia (posteroanterior and lateral views) and check the reduction of any fracture. When passing the intramedullary guidewire, reamers and nail, the knee needs to be flexed over some folded drapes (Figure 84). When locking distally the knee is extended and the tibia is raised up on the drapes and stabilised by an assistant so as to allow clear, unhindered horizontal beam lateral imaging. The theatre set-up is similar to tibial nailing with traction (see above).

Considerations

- Ensure that any pressure areas are well-padded: the occiput, the sacral area, the heels.
- A thigh tourniquet may be used for operations on the leg (but not for intramedullary nailing).
- Drape the leg free to allow full hip, knee and ankle movement.

Surgical approaches

Anterior (freehand intramedullary nailing of the tibia)

Anteromedial   Posterolateral

Anterolateral   Approach to the fibula

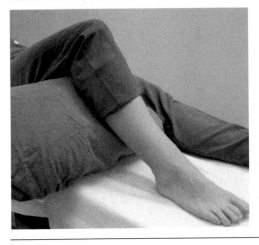

FIG. 84 **Position for freehand tibial intramedullary nailing. Folded drapes under the knee help maintain the position**

Leg (tibia and fibula)

Lateral position

(Figure 85)

- True lateral position on a standard operating table (operative side uppermost)
- Position a padded post against the anterior pelvis
- Position a padded lumbar support against the lumbar spine
- Rest the head on a suitable support (e.g. a pillow or a head ring)
- Flex the knees to relieve tension of the sciatic nerves.

Considerations

- Ensure that the patient is in a stable, well-supported position.
- Ensure that the lower arm is free and not being compressed under the patient's body.
- Support the head sufficiently to keep the neck in a neutral position.
- Ensure that any pressure areas are well-padded: the areas under the post and the lumbar support, the greater trochanter and the lateral malleolus of the lower leg, the medial malleolus of the upper leg.
- Place a pillow between the knees.
- A thigh tourniquet may be used.
- Drape the leg free to allow full hip, knee and ankle movement.
- The surgeon usually stands behind the patient during surgery.

Surgical approaches

Anterolateral

Posterolateral

Approach to the fibula

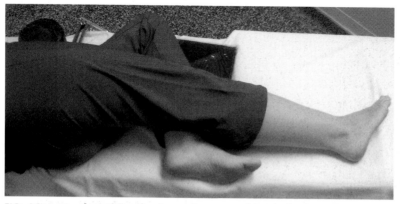

FIG. 85 **Lateral position for lateral approaches to the leg and ankle**

Ankle

Supine position

(Figures 86 and 87)

- Supine position on a standard operating table (may need to be radiolucent)
- Approaches to the medial malleolus: the leg naturally lies in slight external rotation when a patient is supine. To increase external rotation, the figure-of-4 position may be used (Figure 88)
- Approaches to the lateral malleolus: place a sandbag under the buttock to help internally rotate the leg. The access may be improved further by placing a side support against the opposite iliac crest and then tilting the table 20–30° towards the opposite side.

Considerations

- Ensure that any pressure areas are well-padded: the occiput, the sacral area, the heels.
- A thigh tourniquet may be used.
- Drape the leg free to allow full hip, knee and ankle movement.

Surgical approaches

Anterior approach to the distal tibia

Medial malleolus (anteromedial and posteromedial approaches)

Lateral malleolus (lateral approach to the distal fibula)

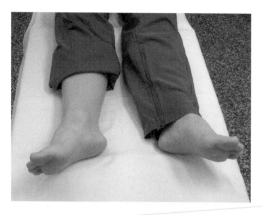

FIG. 86 **Leg lying externally rotated (medial approach to the ankle)**

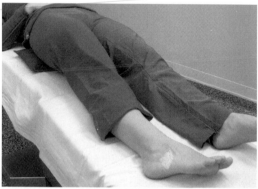

FIG. 87 **Leg internally rotated with a sandbag placed under the buttock (lateral approach to the ankle)**

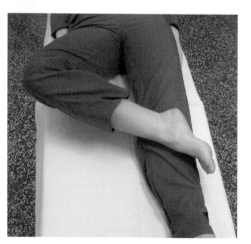

FIG. 88 **Figure-of-4 position (medial approach to the ankle)**

Ankle

Lateral position

(Figures 89 and 90)

- True lateral position on a standard operating table
- Position a padded post against the anterior pelvis
- Position a padded lumbar support against the lumbar spine
- Rest the head on a suitable support (e.g. a pillow or a head ring)
- Flex the knees to relieve tension of the sciatic nerves
- Approaches to the medial malleolus: the operative side is nearest the table and the upper leg is flexed to expose the medial aspect of the lower ankle (Figure 89).
- Approaches to the lateral malleolus: the operative side is uppermost (Figure 90).

The lateral position should not be used if access to both sides of the ankle is required.

Considerations

- Ensure that the patient is in a stable, well-supported position.
- Ensure that the lower arm is free and not being compressed under the patient's body.
- Support the head sufficiently to keep the neck in a neutral position.
- Ensure that any pressure areas are well-padded: the areas under the post and the lumbar support, the greater trochanter and the lateral malleolus of the lower leg, the medial malleolus of the upper leg.
- Place a pillow between the knees.
- A thigh tourniquet may be used.
- Drape the leg free to allow full hip, knee and ankle movement.
- The surgeon usually stands behind the patient during surgery.

Surgical approaches

Medial malleolus (anteromedial and posteromedial approaches)

Lateral malleolus (lateral approach to the distal fibula)

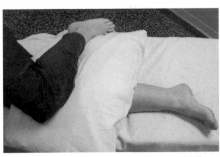

FIG. 89 **Lateral position (contralateral side uppermost) for medial approaches to the ankle**

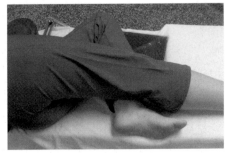

FIG. 90 **Lateral position for lateral approaches to the leg and ankle**

Ankle

Prone position

(Figure 91)

- Transfer the patient on to the operating table in the prone position. This requires rolling the patient from the supine position on to the arms of three or more assistants, who then lift the patient on to the operating table
- In the prone position the patient must have their chest and pelvis supported so as to allow free movement of the abdomen. This may be achieved by lifting the patient on to a special mattress (e.g. the Montreal mattress; see Figure 101)
- Rest the head on a suitable support (e.g. a pillow or a head ring)
- Abduct the shoulders 90° and flex the elbows 90° so that the arms lie supported on a suitable arm board (move the arms through into position from the side in a front crawl swimming motion)
- Place a pillow or a Rhys-Davies exsanguinator under the legs (shins) to flex the knees slightly and relieve tension on the sciatic nerves. Knee flexion will also lift the feet clear of the operating table and allow ankle movement. Alternatively, hang the feet over the end of the operating table.

Considerations

- Ensure that any pressure areas are well-padded: the knees, the pelvis, the external genitalia, the chest, the arms, the forehead.
- Pad and tape the eyes.
- A thigh tourniquet may be used.
- Drape the arm free to allow full shoulder and elbow movement.

Surgical approaches

Posterior   Posteromedial (Achilles tendon)

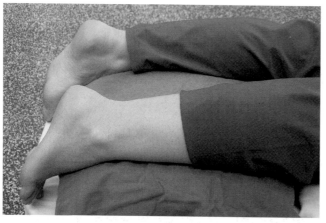

FIG. 91 **Prone position. The legs are supported with the knees flexed and the feet hanging freely**

Foot

Supine position

(Figures 92 and 93)

- Supine position on a standard operating table (may need to be radiolucent)
- Dorsomedial approaches. The leg naturally lies in slight external rotation when a patient is supine (see Figure 86). To increase external rotation, the figure-of-4 position may be used (see Figure 88)
- Lateral and anterolateral approaches to the hindfoot, and dorsolateral approaches to the mid-foot and forefoot. Place a sandbag under the buttock to help internally rotate the leg (see Figure 87). The access may be improved further by placing a side support against the opposite iliac crest and then tilting the table 20–30° towards the opposite side
- Dorsal approaches to the midfoot and forefoot. Flex the knee so that the foot lies with its sole on the table (plantigrade) (Figure 92). This position may be maintained by placing one or more pillows behind the knee
- Plantar approaches (Figure 93). Sit at the end of the table with the table raised. The table may also be tilted head-down (Trendelenburg position).

Considerations

- Ensure that any pressure areas are well-padded: the occiput, the sacral area, the heels.
- A thigh tourniquet may be used.
- Drape the leg free to allow full hip, knee and ankle movement.

Surgical approaches

Anterolateral approach to the hindfoot

Lateral approach to the hindfoot

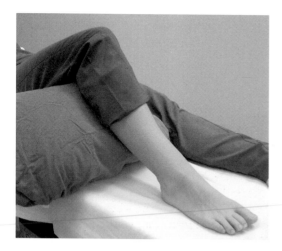

FIG. 92 **Foot supported in a plantigrade position using folded drapes under the knee**

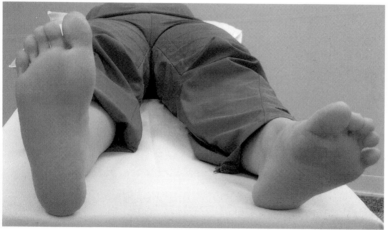

FIG. 93 **Plantar aspect of the foot. A Trendelenburg (head-down) position may be helpful**

Spine

Cervical spine

Supine position

(Figures 94 and 95)

- Supine position on a standard operating table
- Ensure the table break is underneath the lumbosacral area
- Wedge a small sandbag (or a litre bag of fluid) between the scapulae to help extend the neck slightly
- Laterally flex the neck away from the side to be operated on, resting the head on a suitable support (e.g. a head ring). Be careful not to flex the neck excessively as this would risk a traction injury to the brachial plexus
- Elevate the head of the table 30–45° to reduce venous pressure (and thus decrease bleeding) and to allow blood to drain from the operative field
- Flex the knees (e.g. over pillows) to relieve any tension of the sciatic nerves.

Considerations

- Ensure that any pressure areas are well-padded: the occiput, the sacral area, the heels.
- Pad and tape the eyes.
- Place each arm at the patient's side.

Surgical approaches

Anterior

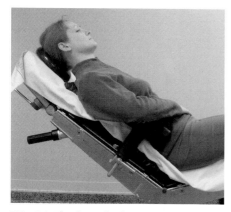

FIG. 94 **The beach-chair position**

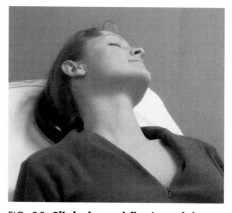

FIG. 95 **Slight lateral flexion of the neck away from the side to be operated on. The head is rested on a suitable support**

Cervical spine

Prone position

(Figure 96)

- Transfer the patient on to the operating table in the prone position. This requires rolling the patient from the supine position on to the arms of three or more assistants, who then lift the patient on to the operating table
- In the prone position the patient must have their chest and pelvis supported so as to allow free movement of the abdomen. This may be achieved by lifting the patient on to a special mattress (e.g. the Montreal mattress; Figure 101) or frame (e.g. the Railton–Hall frame)
- Rest the head on a suitable support (e.g. a pillow or a head ring) so that the neck flexes slightly, thus opening up the interspinous spaces (Figure 97)
- Abduct the shoulders 90° and flex the elbows 90° so that the arms lie supported on a suitable arm board (move the arms through into position from the side in a front crawl swimming motion).

Considerations

- Ensure that any pressure areas are well-padded: the knees, the pelvis, the external genitalia, the chest, the arms, the forehead.
- Pad and tape the eyes.
- Flex the knees slightly (e.g. over a pillow) to relieve tension on the sciatic nerves.

Surgical approaches

Posterior

Alternative

A posterior approach to the cervical spine may also be performed with the patient positioned seated upright with the head held in a special head support. In this position, venous bleeding is reduced, but air embolisation may occur.

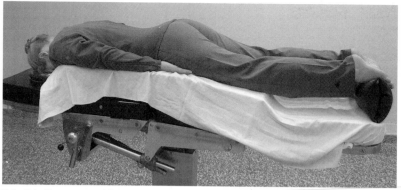

FIG. 96 **Prone position**

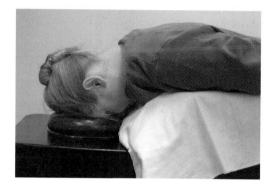

FIG. 97 **Prone position. The head is supported on a gel head ring to allow some neck flexion**

Thoracic spine

Prone position

(Figure 98)

- Transfer the patient on to the operating table in the prone position. This requires rolling the patient from the supine position on to the arms of three or more assistants, who then lift the patient on to the operating table
- In the prone position the patient must have their chest and pelvis supported so as to allow free movement of the abdomen. This may be achieved by lifting the patient on to a special mattress (e.g. the Montreal mattress) or frame (e.g. the Railton–Hall frame)
- Rest the head on a suitable support (e.g. a pillow or a head ring)
- Abduct the shoulders 90° and flex the elbows 90° so that the arms lie supported on a suitable arm board (move the arms through into position from the side in a front crawl swimming motion).

Considerations

- Ensure that any pressure areas are well-padded: the knees, the pelvis, the external genitalia, the chest, the arms, the forehead.
- Pad and tape the eyes.
- The arms are best positioned on an arm board with the shoulders abducted 90° and the elbows flexed 90°.
- Flex the knees slightly (e.g. over a pillow) to relieve tension on the sciatic nerves.

> ### Surgical approaches
>
> Posterior
>
> Posterolateral

Thoracic spine

Lateral position

(Figure 99)

- True lateral position on a standard operating table
- Position a padded post against the anterior pelvis
- Position a padded lumbar support against the lumbar spine
- Rest the head on a suitable support (e.g. a pillow or a head ring)
- Forward flex the ipsilateral arm 90° and rest it on an arm-rest.

Considerations

- Ensure that the patient is in a stable, well-supported position.
- Ensure that the lower arm is free and not being compressed under the patient's body.

- Support the head sufficiently to keep the neck in a neutral position.
- Ensure that any pressure areas are well-padded: the axilla of the lower arm, the areas under the post and the lumbar support, the greater trochanter and the lateral malleolus of the lower leg, the medial malleolus of the upper leg.
- Place a pillow between the knees.
- Flex the knees to relieve tension on the sciatic nerves.
- The surgeon stands behind the patient.

Surgical approaches

Anterolateral thoracotomy

Thoracoabdominal

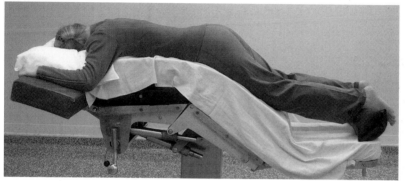

FIG. 98 **Prone position on a Montreal mattress. Note the relaxed arms and the flexed knees**

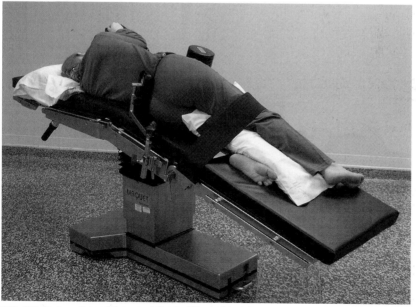

FIG. 99 **Lateral position, with a pillow positioned between the knees**

Lumbar spine

Prone position

(Figures 100 and 101)

- Transfer the patient on to the operating table in the prone position. This requires rolling the patient from the supine position on to the arms of three or more assistants, who then lift the patient on to the operating table
- In the prone position the patient must have their chest and pelvis supported so as to allow free movement of the abdomen. This may be achieved by lifting the patient on to a special mattress (e.g. the Montreal mattress) or frame (e.g. the Railton–Hall frame)
- Rest the head on a suitable support (e.g. a pillow or a head ring)
- Abduct the shoulders 90° and flex the elbows 90° so that the arms lie supported on a suitable arm board (move the arms through into position from the side in a front crawl swimming motion).

Montreal mattress (Figure 101): a shaped mattress with a central cut-out for the abdomen so that the abdomen can lie free, which allows venous drainage into the inferior vena cava and thus reduces venous plexus filling around the spinal cord.

Railton–Hall frame: a frame with four hinged pads that support the chest and pelvis in the prone position, allowing the abdomen to lie free.

Considerations

- Ensure that any pressure areas are well-padded: the knees, the pelvis, the external genitalia, the chest, the arms, the forehead.
- Pad and tape the eyes.
- The arms are best positioned on an arm board with the shoulders abducted 90° and the elbows flexed 90°. The axillae must be free.
- Flex the knees slightly (e.g. over a pillow) to relieve tension on the sciatic nerves.

> ### Surgical approaches
>
> Posterior

Lumbar spine

Lateral position

(Figure 102)

- True lateral position on a standard operating table
- Position a padded post against the anterior pelvis
- Position a padded lumbar support against the thoracic spine
- Rest the head on a suitable support (e.g. a pillow or a head ring)
- Flex the hips to flex the lumbar spine and open up the interspinous spaces

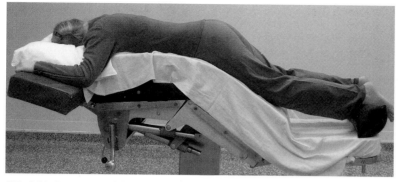

FIG. 100 **Prone position on a Montreal mattress. Note the relaxed arms and the flexed knees**

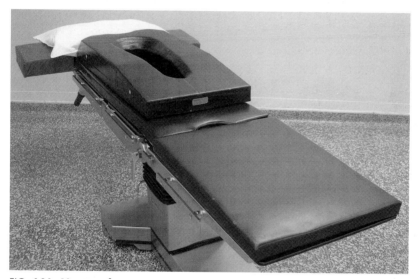

FIG. 101 **Montreal mattress**

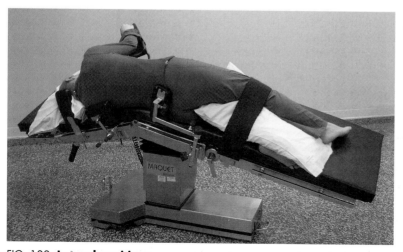

FIG. 102 **Lateral position**

- Jack-knife the table to laterally flex the lumbar spine and so open up the intervertebral spaces further on the upper side. The affected spinal level should be positioned over the table break.

Considerations

- Ensure that the patient is in a stable, well-supported position.
- Ensure that the lower arm is free and not being compressed under the patient's body.
- Support the head sufficiently to keep the neck in a neutral position.
- Ensure that any pressure areas are well-padded: the areas under the post and the lumbar support, the greater trochanter and the lateral malleolus of the lower leg, the medial malleolus of the upper leg.
- Place a pillow between the knees.
- Flex the knees to relieve tension on the sciatic nerves.
- The surgeon stands behind the patient.

Surgical approaches

Posterior

Lumbar spine

Semi-lateral position

- Semi-lateral position on a standard operating table: the patient should be at 45°, halfway between a supine and a true lateral position. The affected side is uppermost
- Keep the patient in position, either by bolstering the back (hips to shoulders) with sandbags or by placing an angled lumbar support against the lumbar spine.

Considerations

- Ensure that the patient is in a stable, well-supported position.
- Ensure that the lower arm is free and not being compressed under the patient's body.
- Support the head sufficiently to keep the neck in a neutral position.
- Ensure that any pressure areas are well-padded: the areas under the lumbar support, the greater trochanter and the lateral malleolus of the lower leg, the medial malleolus of the upper leg.
- Place a pillow between the knees.
- Flex the knees to relieve tension on the sciatic nerves.

Surgical approaches

Anterolateral (retroperitoneal) approach to the lumbar spine

Supine position

- Supine position on a standard operating table.

Considerations

- Ensure that any pressure areas are well-padded: the occiput, the sacral area, the heels.

Surgical approaches

Anterior (transperitoneal) approach to the lumbar spine

Appendix   Positions and approaches

Region	Patient position	Surgical approaches
General surgery		
Abdomen	Dorsal recumbent	Laparotomy; laparoscopic surgery
Perineum	Lithotomy	Abdominal-perineal excision of rectum; endoscopic urological procedures; genitourinary procedures; peri-anal procedures
	Lloyd-Davies	Anterior resection of rectum; genitourinary procedures; pelvic surgery; laparoscopic upper gastrointestinal surgery
	Jack-knife	Anus and rectum; coccyx; thoracolumbar spinal surgery; adrenal surgery
	Knee–chest (lateral or prone)	Sigmoidoscopy
Kidney	Lateral kidney	Nephrectomy; adrenal; aorta; lumbar sympathetic trunk
Vascular	Neck or thyroid	Carotid arterial surgery
	Supine	Aortic aneurysm surgery; iliac arterial surgery; axillo-femoral bypass
	Supine (knee flexed)	Femoro-popliteal bypass
	Supine (arm table)	Forearm arterio-venous fistula
	Trendelenburg	Varicose vein surgery
Head & neck	Neck or thyroid	Thyroid; neck dissection; parotid gland surgery; carotid arterial surgery
Breast	Supine (arm board)	Breast surgery (including axillary dissection); breast reconstruction
Thorax	Supine	Median sternotomy
	Lateral	Lateral thoracotomy
Orthopaedics		
Shoulder	Beach-chair	Anterior (deltopectoral); anterolateral (coronal and parasagittal approaches); lateral (deltoid-splitting)
	Lateral	Posterior
Arm (humerus & elbow)	Prone (arm table)	Posterior (triceps-splitting)
	Lateral (arm over rest)	Posterior (triceps-splitting)
	Supine (arm over chest)	Posterior (humerus and elbow); medial (elbow)

Region	Patient position	Surgical approaches
	Supine (arm table)	Anterior and anterolateral (humerus and elbow); medial (elbow); lateral (humerus and elbow); posterolateral (Kocher–elbow)
Forearm	Supine (arm table) – pronated forearm	Posterolateral (radius); direct medial (ulna)
	– supinated forearm	Anterior (Henry – radius)
	Supine (arm over chest)	Direct medial (ulna); posterior (radius)
Wrist & hand	Supine (arm table) – pronated forearm	Dorsal approaches
	– supinated forearm	Volar approaches
Pelvis	Supine	Anterior (iliac crest)
Hip	Lateral	Direct lateral/transgluteal (Hardinge); posterior
	Supine	Direct lateral/transgluteal (Hardinge); anterolateral (Watson-Jones); anterior (Smith-Petersen); ilioinguinal; medial
Thigh (femur)	Supine (with traction)	Lateral
	Supine (without traction)	Lateral; anteromedial (distal femur); posterolateral (distal femur)
	Lateral (with traction)	Lateral
	Lateral (without traction)	Lateral; posterolateral (distal femur)
Knee	Supine	Anterior; medial; lateral
	Supine (arthroscopy)	Valgus (medial compartment); figure-of-4 (lateral compartment)
	Supine (cruciate ligament surgery)	Anterior
Leg (tibia & fibula)	Supine (with traction)	Anterior
	Supine (without traction)	Anterior; anterolateral; posterolateral
Ankle	Supine	Anterior; anteromedial; posteromedial; lateral
	Prone	Posterior and posteromedial (Achilles tendon)
Foot	Supine (knee extended)	Plantar and dorsal approaoches
	Supine (foot plantigrade)	Dorsal approaches
Cervical spine	Supine	Anterior
	Prone	Posterior

Region	Patient position	Surgical approaches
Thoracic spine	Lateral	Anterolateral thoracotomy; thoracoabdominal
	Prone	Posterior; posterolateral
Lumbar spine	Lateral	Posterior
	Semi-lateral	Thoracoabdominal; anterior retroperitoneal
	Prone	Posterior
	Supine	Anterior (trans-peritoneal)